Psychopharmacology Demystified

Leonard Lichtblau,

PhD

Associate Professor
Department of Experimental and Clinical Pharmacology
College of Pharmacy
University of Minnesota

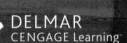 **DELMAR**
CENGAGE Learning

Australia • Brazil • Japan • Korea • Mexico • Singapore • Spain • United Kingdom • United States

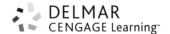

**Psychopharmacology Demystified,
First Edition**
Leonard Lichtblau

Vice President, Career and Professional
Editorial: Dave Garza

Director of Learning Solutions: Matthew Kane

Senior Acquisitions Editor: Maureen Rosener

Managing Editor: Marah Bellegarde

Senior Product Manager: Patricia Gaworecki

Editorial Assistant: Samantha Miller

Vice President, Career and Professional
Marketing: Jennifer Baker

Marketing Director: Wendy E. Mapstone

Senior Marketing Manager: Michele McTighe

Marketing Coordinator: Scott Chrysler

Production Director: Carolyn Miller

Production Manager: Andrew Crouth

Senior Content Project Manager: James Zayicek

Senior Art Director: Jack Pendleton

Production Service: Pre-PressPMG

For product information and technology assistance, contact us at
Cengage Learning Customer & Sales Support, 1-800-354-9706

For permission to use material from this text or product,
submit all requests online at **cengage.com/permissions.**
Further permissions questions can be e-mailed to
permissionrequest@cengage.com

Library of Congress Control Number: 2010922231

ISBN-13: 978-1-435-42787-7

ISBN-10: 1-4354-2787-4

Delmar
5 Maxwell Drive
Clifton Park, NY 12065-2919
USA

Cengage Learning is a leading provider of customized learning solutions with office locations around the globe, including Singapore, the United Kingdom, Australia, Mexico, Brazil, and Japan. Locate your local office at:
international.cengage.com/region

Cengage Learning products are represented in Canada by Nelson Education, Ltd.

For your lifelong learning solutions, visit **delmar.cengage.com**

Visit our corporate website at **cengage.com**

Printed in the United States of America
1 2 3 4 5 6 7 14 13 12 11 10

FLAME has many meanings. It can be a brilliant light, a streak of color, an intense passion, or a sweetheart. Bobbi, my late wife, was all of these to me. She was the flame whose radiance lit up my life and allowed me to see the world. She was my first and only sweetheart, a woman full of life and overflowing with passion, both to be right and to do right. She was a role model of what humanity is supposed to be about. She both loved life and lived life.

When I met her, so long ago, at age 21, she had a shock of pure white hair running along her brow, a sign of where God's tears of joy landed upon her, seeing how beautiful she was. My Bobbi brought lightness into every room she entered and into every life she touched.

Without Bobbi's support and her confidence in me, this project would not have happened. It is to her memory that I dedicate this book. Bobbi's flame shone brightly but oh so briefly upon the world and we are all a little less for her absence today.

Bobbi Lichtblau (1950–2007)

TABLE OF CONTENTS

PREFACE

The preface of a textbook is where the author gives you his or her lofty, dignified and, often, altruistic reasons for writing the book they hope you will purchase. My reasons are, by contrast, mundane and uncomplicated; I accepted a challenge or bet and lost (or won, actually).

Three years ago my colleague Merrie Kaas, DNSc, RN, CS, and I, in the University of Minnesota School of Nursing, had two months to prepare an online psychopharmacology course for advanced practice nursing students, and I wouldn't stop whining about the limited choices of textbooks we could use for the course. What bothered me to no end was that the available psychopharmacology texts were either weighty tomes written by MD-PhDs for MD-PhDs or they were written by authors who seemed to think that impugning the intelligence of *their* potential audience (rhymes with mummies) would get students to flock to college bookstores and shell over hard-earned cash for overly simplified explanations of truly complex phenomena.

What was needed, I felt, was a book that communicated our current understanding of mental illnesses and the drugs used to treat those illnesses, but written using language intelligible by college-educated students pursuing a career in nursing and/or clinical psychology. On top of that, it should be FUN to read. Fed up, Merrie challenged me to put up or shut up and write my own content if I thought I could do better. This book is the result of that challenge.

For each section of the psychopharmacology course, I was responsible for assembling the scientific evidence sections while Merrie addressed the other essential elements that allow mental health professionals to make rational treatment decisions for the patient, and to maximize the chance of a successful therapeutic outcome (*Model for Psychopharmacotherapeutic Management*, developed by Merrie Kaas). The course was a tremendous success and I was encouraged by our students to assemble my contributions into a textbook and get it published. So, voila, *Psychopharmacology Demystified*, at your service.

PEDAGOGICAL ELEMENTS

This book does not fit the standard definition or composition of a textbook. Unlike traditional pharmacology and psychology texts, it does not offer identically organized chapters with consistent section headers. Each chapter in this textbook stands on its own, with a unique *je ne sais quoi* (that's French for a pleasing characteristic that is difficult to describe—and it makes me sound so clever). Moreover, *Psychopharmacology Demystified* is not filled with copious quantities of pharmacokinetic and pharmacodynamic factoids or with exhaustive lists of every drug used to treat every disease or illness (If you are looking that level of detail, purchase Delmar's *Nurse's Drug Handbook*.)

Instead, *Psychopharmacology Demystified* is filled with stories (read about the first bad acid-trip) and fun-facts (carbon monoxide is a neurotransmitter; the first clinically useful antidepressants were developed by the Allies from leftover chemicals used by the Germans to fuel the rockets that showered over England during WW II). The stories are designed to capture your attention and keep you reading through the tedious material (Sorry, I can't entirely eliminate it). Each chapter begins with a quote (because I love quotes) and often with a personal vignette, written by a patient or family member (to remind you that, although the book focuses on illnesses and drugs, ultimately it is about people.) This book is written for you—the student—the one who needs to use the information. You may find that this book is a little like its author, rumpled, disheveled, irreverent, and fun to be around (LOL).

A word of warning: Don't buy this textbook if all you want are the answers. You won't find them here. I believe an exceptional textbook and a first-class higher education is one that not only gives you some answers, but more importantly, it gives you new questions. But don't panic! Answers and rationales are provided for all end-of-chapter review questions and are located in the Answer Key at the back of the book.

"Model for Psychopharmacotherapeutic Management" developed by Merrie Kaas.

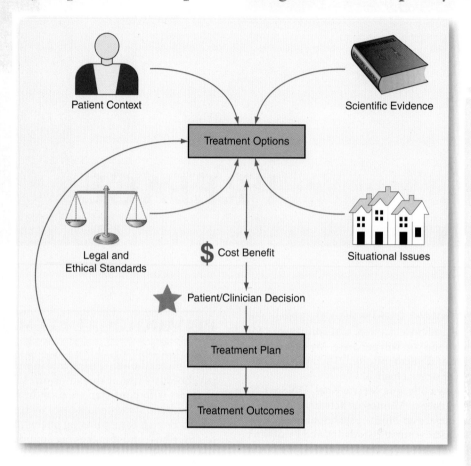

So, if you actually have gotten this far and read this entire Preface, and perhaps enjoy the book, please send me an e-mail (len@umn.edu) and let me know. I'll even write back to you. Enjoy![1]

Len Lichtblau, PhD
Associate Professor
College of Pharmacy and School of Nursing
University of Minnesota

---

[1] "Human salvation lies in the hands of the creatively maladjusted." —Martin Luther King Jr.

ACKNOWLEDGMENTS

I wish to acknowledge the contributions of my editors at Cengage; Maureen Rosener, who found me; Patty Gaworecki, who kept me on a straight path, and Katherine Kraines, who made my book more readable. I, too, thank Pradhiba Kannaiyan and the production staff at Pre-PressPMG who brought life to my ideas and to the countless others at Cengage who contributed to the success of this endeavor.

I want to thank my colleague Merrie Kaas at the University of Minnesota School of Nursing for issuing me a challenge I didn't back away from and for being there for me when I needed her. I would be remiss not to thank two of my dearest friends, Jill Marks and Cathy Bloomfield, both of whom are clinical psychologists and both of whom gave me the courage to face dark times and move forward, not just with this book, but with life in general. You will always be in my heart.

I also need to acknowledge "anonymous," for the personal vignettes they contributed to the beginning of most chapters. A real patient or family member wrote each vignette. They, as one, wanted me to remind health care professionals that you are treating people, not diseases. They felt their stories at the start of each chapter would help and so, as difficult as it was for some, they wrote their stories.

Lastly, there is my family to thank, both those born into it—including my sons Andy and Danny—and those who have moved into this circle by assimilation. "They" say you can pick your friends but you can't pick your relatives. I disagree. Over the years I have chosen a select group of dear friends and decided they are my family, and so it is. I want to thank my family for their boundless love, their warmhearted compassion, and for their unflagging support through the bad times and the good. God bless.[1]

Len Lichtblau

---

[1] "Honest criticism is hard to take, particularly from a relative, a friend, an acquaintance, or a stranger." —Franklin P. Jones

REVIEWERS

Deanah Alexander, RN, CNS, MSN
Instructor
West Texas A&M University
Canyon, Texas

Lora Humphrey Beebe, PhD, PMHNP-BC
Assistant Professor
University of Tennessee, College of Nursing
Knoxville, Tennessee

Yoriko Kozuki, PhD, PMHNP-BC, ARNP
Associate Professor
University of Washington
Seattle, Washington

Barbara Jones Warren, PhD, RN, CNS, CS
Associate Professor
Ohio State University, College of Nursing
Columbus, Ohio

Editor
Katherine L. Kraines

CHAPTER 1

Neuroanatomy and Neurophysiology

"Yes, Agassiz does recommend authors to eat fish, because the phosphorus in it makes brain. So far you are correct. But I cannot help you to a decision about the amount you need to eat—at least, not with certainty. If the specimen composition you send is about your fair usual average, I should judge that a couple of whales would be all you would want for the present. Not the largest kind, but simply good middling-sized whales."

MARK TWAIN

INTRODUCTION

It has taken a long time for the medical community and society in general to begin to comprehend the complex biology of mental illness. In the past, people struggling with mental health issues were generally misunderstood and frequently viewed as having a personality defect, or worse. These patients were often placed out of sight or were forced to live on the margins of society, suffering the consequences of mental illness, while both patients and their families struggled with the fear and shame that often accompanied the disease. But in the past 150 years, increasing research, new drugs, and a better understanding of the biology and chemistry of mental illness have lead to significant changes in the medical and societal treatment of those with mental health issues. It is important to understand that depression, bipolar disorder, schizophrenia, generalized anxiety disorder, or other such conditions are not due to character weaknesses, cannot be caught from other people, and are not—as was once thought—induced by the phases of the moon. Mental illness is due to neurochemical dysfunction(s) in specific areas of the brain.

This book discusses diseases and illnesses that affect the brain and the drugs used to treat these disorders. Throughout this text, the anatomical focus (or foci) of an illness (neuroanatomy), the normal function of the areas affected (neurophysiology), and the neurochemical targets for drug action (neuropharmacology) are discussed. This chapter provides some of the basic language needed to understand the concepts that are presented.

Think of the central nervous system as a house, made up of several floors with numerous rooms on each level. The relatively brief neuroanatomy section entitled The Brain describes the floors of the house (brainstem, diencephalon, and cerebrum) and the rooms on each floor (cerebral cortex, amygdala, cerebellum, etc.) with additional neuroanatomical details addressed as needed (Figure 1-1). In the house, there are multiple ways in which the rooms can be connected to each other and to a host of central control systems that may include electrical wiring, plumbing, telephone lines, and cable. Often, the systems that go into and out of a room

indicate the room's function. For example, a small room with a significant amount of plumbing and some electrical connections is likely to be a bathroom. Make the room larger and add more wiring and it is probably the kitchen. This is also true of the central nervous system, specifically the different areas of the brain. The relative size, various control systems, and "wiring" or interconnections between each part of the brain provide important clues to each area's function(s) and role. The Neurophysiology Overview later in this chapter discusses the "wiring" of the brain and the chemicals used in the nervous system to pass information from cell-to-cell and tissue-to-tissue.

In general, many human diseases and illnesses can be cured by surgery or successfully treated with drugs (synthetic or natural), and in managing mental illness drugs often play a key role in the treatment regimen. Now, a full decade into the twenty-first century, it is clear that the basis of mental illness is biological (Society for Neuroscience, 2008). That is, the symptoms are due to known or unknown chemical imbalance(s) somewhere in the brain. Psychoactive drugs act in the brain to correct these neurochemical imbalances, thereby reducing or eliminating abnormal behavior. This chapter covers the process of neurotransmission and describes the action of key brain neurotransmitters that are associated with normal brain function and mental illness, and that are responsible for the clinical efficacy of psychoactive drugs.

When choosing to use a particular tool with a patient— time, talk, herbs, drugs, or surgery—it is important to understand the tool's nuances and how it can be used most effectively. If a drug is used, it is vital to know how the drug works, what it can be used for, and when it should *not* be used. It is prudent to remember that information that seems definitive today can quickly change and expand as new research provides insights into the brain. Although much has been learned about how the brain functions, there is still much to discover. The fact is "We don't know what we don't know."

TERMS

Psychopharmacology is a branch of pharmacology that examines the effects of drugs on cognition, emotion, and behavior. How do drugs accomplish this? For some drugs, there are good answers, while in other cases, although the drugs work, it is still not known how they work. A basic tenet of pharmacology is that drugs do not create new functions; rather, they alter existing functions to correct (or, in some cases, create) imbalances (DiPiro, Talbert, Yee, Matzke, & Wells, 2008).

Physiology is the science of the normal functions and phenomena of living organisms (Widmaier, Raff, & Strang, 2008). Limiting this science to the workings of the brain falls under the classification of neurophysiology (which covers the entire nervous system). The brain is not a homogenous sack of indistinguishable cells with each cell capable of controlling any neuronal function in any part of the body. In fact, the brain is highly complex and organized hierarchically (Oregon Public Broadcasting). It is regionalized, sub-regionalized, and sub-sub-regionalized, with each region regulating different functions (vision, speech, movement, memory, emotion) or even different aspects of the same function (an object's color, shape, distance, and identity).

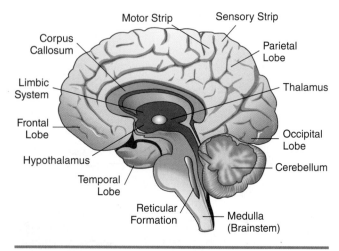

FIGURE 1-1 General overview of key neuroanatomical structures in the brain.

BOX 1-1
BRAIN TRIVIA QUIZ

1. What is approximate weight of the average human brain?[1]
   a. 0.75 pound
   b. 1.5 pounds
   c. 3 pounds
   d. 6 pounds

2. Approximately how many neurons are contained in the human brain?[2]
   a. 100 million
   b. 1 billion
   c. 100 billion
   d. 1 trillion

3. A connection between two neurons in the nervous system is known as a synapse. Approximately how many synapses occur in the human brain?[3]
   a. 500,000
   b. 500,000,000
   c. 500,000,000,000
   d. 500,000,000,000,000

4. The part of the brain that makes a person uniquely human is the cerebral cortex, the outermost layer of the brain. What is the average thickness of the human cerebral cortex?[4]
   a. 0.2–0.5 mm (0.007–0.019 in)
   b. 1.5–4.5 mm (0.06–0.18 in)
   c. 4.0–12 mm (0.16–0.47 in)
   d. 20–50 mm (0.79–1.96 in)

[1]The average adult human brain weighs about 3 pounds. Although the brain makes up only about 2% of the body's mass, it uses about 20% of the body's oxygen.

[2]A neuron is a specialized cell within the nervous system that conducts electrical impulses along its processes. It is the wiring network in the nervous system. It is estimated that the human brain contains over 100 billion neurons. The majority of brain cells, however, are glial cells and astrocytes that help maintain the structure of the brain. They outnumber neurons by a factor of 10 (1 trillion glial cells).

[3]The connection between two neurons is known as a synapse. Although most diagrams of a synapse imply that the relationship between the neurons is one-to-one; that is, one neuron innervates only one neuron, in most cases this is far from the truth. In the brain, a single neuron can get input from an average of 5000 other neurons. The effect on that neuron depends on the net number of excitatory and inhibitory inputs. If there are more excitatory than inhibitory inputs the net effect is activation of the neuron.

[4]The part of the brain that makes a person uniquely human lies in less than 1/10 of an inch (~ 3 mm) of the very topmost layer (cerebral cortex) of. It is here that thought, language, reasoning, perception, and personality are controlled.

Neuroanatomy is the scientific study of the anatomical organization of the nervous system (brain, spinal cord, peripheral nerves). To help clinicians make rational decisions as to which psychopharmacological agent is best for a particular clinical situation (depression, for example), it is important to know what brain function is altered and where it is altered. Mental illness is due to a neurochemical (neurotransmitter, NT) imbalance in a particular area or areas of the brain. It is the rare drug than acts in a single location in the body, even when it is clear which NT is perturbed, where in the brain the disruption is occurring, and that the correct drug is chosen to remediate the problem. Most drugs change the NT level throughout the brain, even in areas where its levels may have been normal. Consequently, many drugs have undesirable side effects. It is possible to predict both clinical effectiveness and the potential for adverse effects of a drug by understanding how the drug affects the specific NTs in the brain.

Before reading this chapter, which begins with some neuroanatomy and physiology, try the Brain Trivia Quiz to get a glimpse of the immense complexity of the human brain.

THE NERVOUS SYSTEM

Most living species have two forms of communication between parts of the body. One form of communication is accomplished through chemicals (hormones) that travel from one part of the body to another in the blood. The second form is by neurotransmission, where information is conveyed by an exquisite blend of both electrical and chemical signals (neurotransmitters) via specialized cells known as neurons. This network of neurons, as a whole, is referred to as the nervous system.

THE STRUCTURE OF THE NERVOUS SYSTEM

The human nervous system (Figure 1-2) can be divided into the central nervous system (CNS) and the peripheral nervous system (PNS). Each of these two primary divisions can be further subdivided. The PNS carries sensory (afferent) information about the external environment (heat, cold, pain, color, shape) and internal environment (blood pressure, heartbeat, digestion) to the brain and it carries motor (efferent) signals from the brain to other organs of the body. The motor division is still further divided depending on whether the information conveyed is voluntary (somatic nervous system—moves the hand in response to touching something hot) or involuntary (autonomic nervous system—maintains heartbeat and respiration, even during sleep).

The central nervous system is composed of the brain and spinal cord. While some functions originate in the spinal cord, its chief role is as a physical conduit for getting information to and from the brain and other parts of the body and, to a degree, filtering and fine-tuning the information to improve signal quality.

Over millions of years of evolution, as species evolved from simple unicellular organisms to the incredible complexity of humans, a key element of advancement was the development of a more and more complex neural network and eventually a brain. David J. Linden points out in his book *The Accidental Mind* (Linden, 2008) that as evolution ensued from the reptilian brain to the human brain, when new functions and their associated brain structures were needed they were added to the existing structures. At no

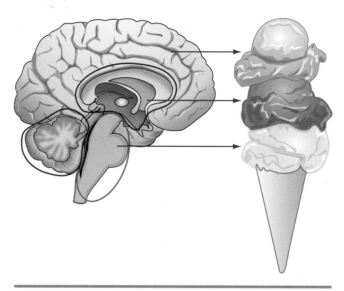

FIGURE 1-3 A three-scoop ice cream cone symbolizing the phylogenetic development of the human brain. Based on Linden (2008).

point was there ever a complete overhaul and redesign of the brain. Consequently, the human brain does not operate as efficiently as it might and there are ancient parts of the brain that humans share with their reptilian ancestors. The oldest brain structures are associated with basic survival needs, such as maintaining respiration, heart rate, and fight-or-flight reactions, whereas the newest structures provide qualities that make humans unique—including conscious-awareness and decision-making. In Linden's analogy, the evolving brain is like a triple-scoop ice cream cone (Figure 1-3), with the bottom scoop (brainstem) common to all species with brains, the second scoop (hypothalamus, thalamus, limbic system, and simple cortex) common among more advanced species such as humans and lower mammals, and the third scoop (a highly structured cortex) that is unique to humans.

The human brain is made up of many parts with each part located in the same place and serving the same function in all humans. Most structures in the brain have been identified and named and have clearly identified functions; the human brain has been studied for hundreds of years, yet there are still some structures whose functions are not fully understood. For example, why do lesions to the insula immediately stop a person's desire to smoke cigarettes (Naqvi, Rudrauf, Damasio, & Bechara, 2007)? There are also many functions whose precise cellular locus (or loci) are not clear, such as how memories are made and stored.

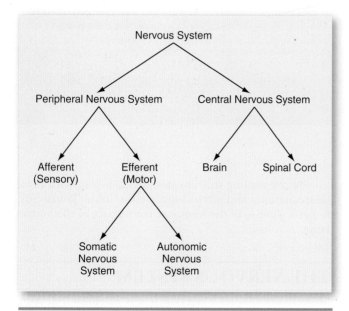

FIGURE 1-2 Bifurcation and rebirfurcation of the nervous system. The human nervous system has two main branches, the central nervous system (composed of the brain and spinal cord) and the peripheral nervous system. The peripheral nervous system has two branches as well: the afferent (sensory) and the efferent (motor) divisions. The efferent component is further subdivided into the somatic (voluntary) and the autonomic (involuntary) divisions.

THE BRAIN

Throughout the brain (Figure 1-4), there are many hundreds of identified and named anatomical structures. This chapter addresses only the major structures of the brain: the cerebrum, diencephalon, cerebellum, and brainstem, although smaller structures (such as the hippocampus, hypothalamus and basal nuclei) are covered in greater depth in this chapter if they are important for understanding later parts of this text, including the areas that are involved in mental illness or are targets for psychoactive drugs.

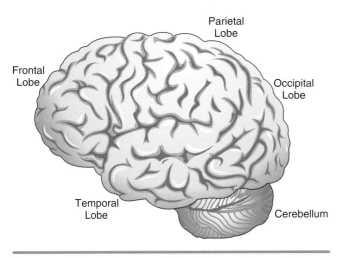

FIGURE 1-4 The four major lobes of the cerebrum and the cerebellum.

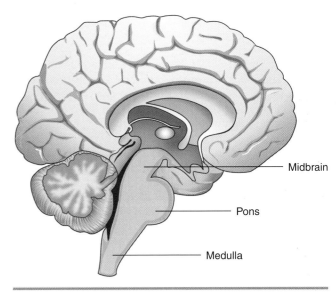

FIGURE 1-5 The medulla, pons, and midbrain.

CLASSIFICATION SYSTEMS

Just as there are many ways to slice a pie, there are a number of classification systems used to describe the major parts of the brain. Four ways of looking at the divisions of the brain are shown in Table 1-1. Row 2 of the table shows the major constituent parts of the brain and is the classification system used in this text.

Although it is a key element in the central nervous system, the spinal cord plays little or no role in mental illness. Thus, the examination of the structure of the brain will begin at the brainstem and end at the cortex.

THE BRAINSTEM

The three principal parts of the brainstem (Figure 1-5) are the midbrain, pons, and medulla. In addition, nuclei are involved in the processing of information from 10 of the 12 cranial nerves that traverse the brainstem. These include peripheral

nerves that innervate muscles, glands, and sensory (e.g., smell, tastes, vision) receptors in the head, as well as thoracic and abdominal organs. Another crucial and fundamental—yet somewhat diffuse—structure in the brainstem is the reticular activating formation and its connection. Together these are referred to as the reticular activating system, a part of the brain responsible for maintaining arousal and wakefulness. In the ice cream cone example, the brainstem is the bottom scoop and is necessary for survival.

The key structures of the brainstem are:

- *Medulla.* This is the lowest level of the brainstem. It lies between the spinal cord and the rest of the brain and is highly involved in regulating many vital body functions including respiration and heart rate. It also contains important centers for reflexes such as sneezing, coughing, and vomiting. In addition, two small round structures, the olives, are needed for balance and coordination, and for

TABLE 1-1 Divisions of the Brain

1	Forebrain				Cerebellum	Brainstem
2	Frontal lobes Temporal lobes Parietal lobes Occipital lobes Corpus collosum	Caudate nucleus Putamen Globus pallidus	Amygdala Hippocampus	Thalamus Hypothalamus	Cerebellum	Midbrain (superior colliculi, inferior colliculi) Pons Medulla oblongota
3	Neocortex	Basal nuclei	Limbic system	Diencephalon	Cerebellum	Brainstem
4	Cerebral Hemispheres			Diencephalon	Cerebellum	Brainstem

modulation of sound impulses from the inner ear. Lastly, key descending motor tracts to skeletal muscles pass through the medulla.

- *Pons.* The pons lies just above the medulla. This area of the brainstem is engaged in some level of motor control and sensory analysis. A portion of the pons helps relay information between the cerebellum and the cerebrum. The nuclei (identifiable masses of neural cell bodies in the brain or spinal cord) for several cranial nerves are found within the pons. In the pons are the sleep and respiratory centers, which, together with the medullary respiratory center, help control respiration.

- *Midbrain.* The main elements of the midbrain are four nuclei that form mounds or hills (colliculi) on the dorsal surface. There are two inferior and two superior colliculi. The inferior colliculi are involved in hearing and in conducting impulses from inner ear structures to the brain. The superior colliculi receive input from the eyes as well as from the skin, the cerebrum, and the inferior colliculi. They also regulate reflexive movement of the eyes and head in response to a host of stimuli. The pathway from the cerebrum to the superior colliculi helps the eyes track moving objects.

  Ascending tracts from the spinal cord to the brain and descending motor pathways from the cerebrum to the spinal cord pass through the midbrain. The midbrain is an important way station for sensory and motor information.

- *Substantia nigra* (Latin for "black substance"). This is another key nucleus located in the midbrain. Its natural pigment allows this area to be visualized microscopically without tissue staining. Cells originating here innervate the basal nuclei in forebrain and help coordinate movement and muscle tone. Degeneration of dopamine (DA)-producing cell bodies in this region is believed to be the root cause of Parkinsonism, a degenerative neurologic disorder. (Key neurotransmitter is DA.)

- *Reticular activating system.* The reticular activating system (RAS) is a series of smaller nuclei spread throughout the brainstem, in both the pons and the medulla. The main function of the RAS is maintaining alertness and motivation. This system is key in sustaining the body's sleep/wake cycle.

  Visual (flashing lights) and auditory (alarm clock) cues as well as mental activities stimulate the RAS to maintain consciousness, sustain attention, and preserve alertness. If the RAS is not stimulated, the person may become drowsy and fall asleep. The RAS is essential in maintaining and fine-tuning cardiovascular and respiratory function in response to the body's demands.

  The degree to which RAS cells innervate higher areas of the brain contributes significantly to a person's ability to focus on certain events, by stimulating some areas of the brain and inhibiting others. The RAS is so important to survival that injury to these areas can lead to coma and death. The reticular activating system is also believed to be a key target in the brain for general anesthetics and sleep medications.

  Neurotransmitters released by neurons whose cell bodies are found in the RAS, and whose axons project throughout the brain, include norepinephrine (NE), serotonin (5-HT), and acetylcholine (ACh). (Key neurotransmitters are NE, 5-HT, and ACh.)

- *Locus ceruleus* (LC, Latin for "the blue spot"). Located at the junction of the pons and midbrain, the locus ceruleus is a key center in the brain for NE-producing neurons that innervate several other areas throughout the brain. (Key neurotransmitter is NE.)

- *Raphe nuclei* (Greek for "seam"). The raphe nuclei are located at the junction of the pons and the medulla. Many of the neurons located here secrete 5-HT and send fibers to innervate the diencephalon and cerebral cortex. Other fibers descend to the spinal cord and may be involved in pain pathways. (Key neurotransmitter is 5-HT.)

THE CEREBELLUM

The literal translation of cerebellum, a structure that looks somewhat like a cauliflower, is "little brain." It is located at the back of the brain, below the occipital lobe of the cerebral cortex and posterior to the pons (Figure 1-6). It is an essential element of the motor control system. The cerebellum is highly interconnected with two other key motor centers in the brain, the motor cortex and the basal nuclei. Despite its size, relative to other "more important" areas of the brain, it contains more neurons than the rest of the brain combined. Over 40 million fibers come to it from the cerebral cortex alone.

Although its role in maintaining motor control functions has been known for a long time, the cerebellum also appears to play a key role in cognitive processes that require precise timing, such as playing a musical instrument, hitting a baseball, or driving a golf ball. The cerebellum helps determine the precise timing sequence for contraction and/or relaxation of multiple skeletal muscles throughout the body, especially when these movements must occur very rapidly and sequentially. Although skeletal muscles are under voluntary control, the high degree of integration among various muscle groups necessary for rapid complex movements requires a high level of control. Feedback from the senses about how the body is

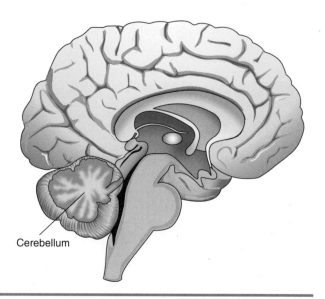

Cerebellum

FIGURE 1-6 The cerebellum lies at the back of the brain, below the occipital lobe of the cerebral cortex and posterior to the pons.

moving in space at any moment is used to finely adjust ongoing movement so that it is fluid, smooth, and well coordinated (for example, the perfectly timed home-run swing of Alex Rodriguez or the graceful golf swing of Tiger Woods). Damage to the cerebellum, unlike injury to other motor areas of the brain, does not result in paralysis. Rather, motor activity becomes less fluid and coordinated.

Although the cerebellum primarily regulates motor activity, it also appears to play some role in learning and memory, particularly for motor functions. It may store some memories of previous movements so that they are executed more effectively in the future. There is also evidence that it may play a role in other aspects of behavior. Some researchers have suggested that damage to the cerebellum may play a role in autism (Hashimoto et al., 1995). The large number of brain-injured soldiers coming home from the wars in Iraq and Afghanistan may provide unprecedented opportunities to study the effects of cerebellar damage.

THE DIENCEPHALON

Although in primitive animals the diencephalon (or interbrain) is a structure distinct from the remainder of the brain, in humans it is so tightly integrated with the cerebrum and the lower parts of the brain that it is difficult to truly demarcate its boundaries. The diencephalon is defined roughly as the structures that surround the third ventricle (fluid-filled cavity) of the brain (Figure 1-7). The two most important structures in the diencephalon are the thalamus and the hypothalamus.

The thalamus (Latin for "inner chamber") is a way station in the brain. Almost all sensory—particularly somatosensory (relating to the perception of sensory stimuli from the skin and internal organs)—information coming in from the spinal cord and lower parts of the brain passes through the thalamus before reaching the cerebrum and other parts of the brain.

These pathways are not just unidirectional; there are also numerous two-way connections between the thalamus and many cortical areas so that much of the information leaving the cerebral cortex passes through the thalamus on its way out. In addition, pathways to and from the cortex and basal nuclei—another region of the brain involved in motor function—also pass through the thalamus.

Among the signals relayed through the thalamus are:

- Somatosensory signals (touch, pressure, pain, temperature, etc.) to appropriate areas of the parietal cortex
- Visual signals to the occipital cortex
- Auditory signals to the superior temporal gyrus of the cortex
- Muscle control signals from the cerebellum and brainstem to the motor cortex and basal nuclei

The hypothalamus, as it name implies, lies below the thalamus. Although relatively small, it controls or regulates numerous and diverse body functions. It is essential in maintaining homeostasis and plays a key role in emotional behavior. The hypothalamus is a unique junction in the brain in which the nervous system and the endocrine system intersect and communicate with each other. The hypothalamus receives and transmits information via neurons and hormones. Neuronal information from higher areas of the brain triggers the hypothalamus to release several hormones. Hypothalamic hormones, rather than entering the general circulation as do other hormones in the body, utilize a specialized series of blood vessels (i.e., portal circulation) to deliver hypothalamic-releasing hormones (or factors) directly to the pituitary gland, which subsequently releases additional hormones into the circulation. Secretion of hormones by the hypothalamus is also regulated by the levels of circulating pituitary hormones as part of a feedback loop.

The hypothalamus regulates specific homeostatic functions that include:

- Blood pressure and heart rate
- Body temperature
- Body water (via thirst and urine output)
- Uterine contractility and milk ejection
- Eating and digestion (hunger, satiety, GI stimulation)
- Hormone secretion from the anterior pituitary via releasing hormones

Behavioral functions of the hypothalamus include:

- General level of activity, rage, fighting
- Tranquility
- Fear and punishment reactions
- Sexual drive

THE LIMBIC SYSTEM

Limbic is Latin for "border." The limbic system (Figure 1-8) is composed of several structures that form the inner border of the cerebrum and the outer border of the diencephalon, surrounding the hypothalamus. Its primary function is to control emotional and behavioral activities.

What structures comprise the limbic system? While this seems like a simple question, it doesn't have a simple answer and over time the answer has shifted. Even today some anatomists include the thalamus and hypothalamus as part of the limbic system while others do not. Additional brain structures

Diencephalon

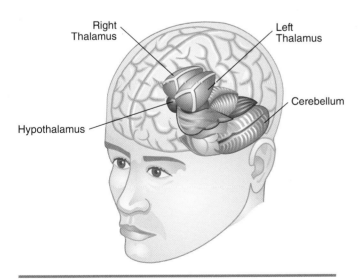

Right Thalamus

Left Thalamus

Cerebellum

Hypothalamus

FIGURE 1-7 **Structures within the diencephalon include the thalamus and the hypothalamus.**

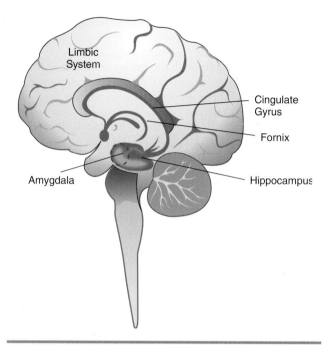

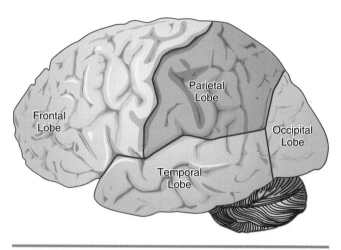

FIGURE 1-9 The four main lobes of the cerebral cortex are shown. These are the frontal, parietal, temporal, and occipital lobes. Below the occipital lobe is the cerebellum (not labeled).

FIGURE 1-8 The limbic system. The two main components of the limbic system are the amygdala and the hippocampus. Other structures include the cingulate gyrus and the fornix. Some anatomists classify the thalamus, hypothalamus and the olfactory cortex as part of the limbic system as well.

that may be considered part of the limbic system are the cingulate gyrus, fornix, mammillary body, pituitary gland, dentate gyrus, and olfactory bulb. Two key structures that everyone agrees are part of the limbic system are the following:

- *Amygdala* (Greek for "almond" or "tonsil"). The amygdala is part of the basal nuclei and it is functionally associated with the limbic system in that it plays a key role in helping people to display appropriate behavior for varying social situations. Injury to the amygdala (located deep inside each anterior temporal lobe) can affect emotion (particularly fear), decision-making, memory, attention, homeostatic processes (heart rate, respiration, etc.—via connections to the hypothalamus) and behavioral responses.
- *Hippocampus* (Greek for "seahorse"). The hippocampus plays a critical role in memory. It receives the sensory information that the cortex has already processed. The hippocampus is the key area of the brain for extended (about a year), but not permanent, memory of facts and events. Damage to the hippocampus will dramatically affect a person's ability to store memories. It also appears to be a key area of the brain affected in patients who are depressed (see Chapter 2) and those with Alzheimer's disease (see Chapter 5).

THE CEREBRUM ✓

The cerebrum (Figure 1-9) is composed of two cerebral hemispheres connected to each other by several bundles of nerve fibers. Two nerve bundles, the corpus callosum and the anterior commissure, connect corresponding points in each hemisphere to ones on the other side. The surface of the cerebrum is highly folded. Each convolution is called a gyrus and the groove between the gyri is a sulcus.

The deepest sulci are referred to as fissures. The longitudinal fissure separates the two hemispheres and the central sulcus extends laterally just about dividing the cerebrum into anterior and posterior halves. These physical markers and two other demarcations, the lateral or sylvian fissure and the parieto-occipital sulcus, help delineate functional elements of the cerebrum.

The advantage of all the folding in the brain is that it allows a larger surface area to exist in a tightly contained solid chamber (the skull). Although the outer, exposed surface of the brain has an area of only 600 cm^2, the entire surface area, including the folds, is several times larger, taking up about 2500 cm^2. While less than 5 mm thick on average, the cerebral cortex contains about 50 to 60 billion neurons and makes about 240 trillion synapses.

The lobes of the cerebrum include:

- Frontal
- Parietal
- Temporal
- Occipital

Each of these lobes has a twin in the right and left hemispheres of the brain.

FRONTAL LOBE

Four primary functions are associated with the frontal lobe of the cerebrum (Figure 1-10):

- *Primary motor cortex.* This area of the cerebrum contains cells of origin for descending motor pathways and is involved in initiating voluntary movements and controlling specific muscles throughout the body, especially those involved in fine movement.
- *Premotor area.* This area is related to the initiation of voluntary movements. This is the section of the brain that stores specific knowledge for controlling skilled movements that have already been learned (playing "Flight of the Bumblebee" in a concert).
- *Broca's area.* This region of the frontal cortex is important for speech and written language. It coordinates movement of the larynx and mouth to produce words. For 95% of all

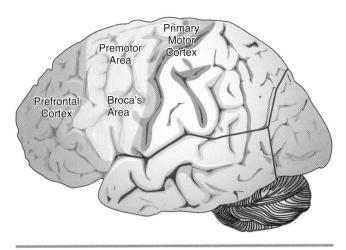

FIGURE 1-10 **Key areas of the frontal lobe of the cortex include the prefrontal cortex, premotor area, Broca's area, and the primary motor cortex.**

people, and in 100% of those who are right-handed, the speech center exists only in the left hemisphere.

- *Prefrontal cortex.* The specific functions of this area are the least well defined of any other region of the cerebrum. This is believed to be the territory in which personality, insight, and foresight originate. Damage to or removal of the prefrontal cortex inhibits/prevents the ability to concentrate for extended periods and interferes with the ability to think through problems.

PARIETAL LOBE

The three key functions associated with these areas of the parietal lobe of the cerebrum (Figure 1-11) are:

- *Somatosensory cortex.* This area is involved in the initial processing of sensory information arriving from sensors throughout the body. These include sensations of touch, pressure, and pain.
- *Parietal lobe association area.* This area is where sensory information arriving in the secondary area has already been processed in deeper brain structures and in the primary

sensory area. This region helps interpret the quality of the signal received (i.e., what is being touched—fur or sandpaper).

- *Wernicke's area.* This section lies at the juncture of the temporal, occipital, and parietal lobes of the cerebral cortex. It is critically involved in the interpretation of language, whether it is external (hearing something said) or internal (thoughts).

TEMPORAL LOBE

These three significant functions are associated with the temporal lobe of the cerebrum (Figure 1-12):

- *Auditory response.* The primary auditory area helps the brain interpret auditory issues such as specific tones and loudness of sounds. The secondary area helps interpret the meaning of spoken words. Both areas play a role in recognizing music.
- *Emotional and visceral responses.* The hippocampus, a part of the limbic system, is folded into the temporal lobe.
- *Learning and memory.* The lower half of the temporal lobe seems to be involved in short-term memory (minutes to weeks).

OCCIPITAL LOBE

The principal function of the occipital lobe of the cerebrum (Figure 1-13) is related to vision. The primary visual area detects light and dark spots, directions of lines, and the borders of objects being observed. The secondary area is involved in interpreting visual information. In other words, the primary visual area helps in seeing the words and images and the secondary area helps it all to make sense.

BASAL NUCLEI (BASAL GANGLIA)

Deep within the cerebrum, below the cerebral lobes, lay several groups of cells known as the basal nuclei (or less precisely, the basal ganglia[5]) (Figure 1-14). The three foremost basal nuclei

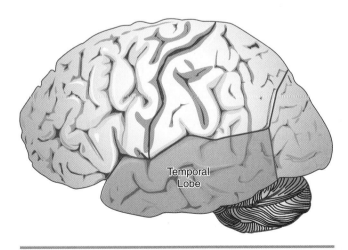

FIGURE 1-12 **The temporal lobe of the cortex.**

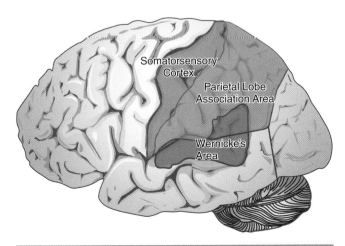

FIGURE 1-11 **Within the parietal lobe are the somatosensory cortex, parietal lobe association area, and Wernicke's area.**

[5]A nucleus is a collection of cell bodies in the central nervous system. In the peripheral nervous system, the term for this is a *ganglion*. Therefore, when talking about a collection of cell bodies in the brain, the more precise term is basal nuclei rather than basal ganglia.

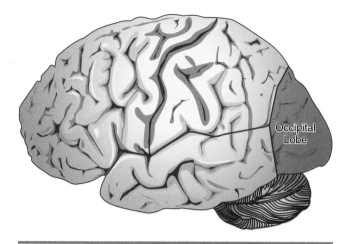

FIGURE 1-13 **The occipital lobe of the cortex.**

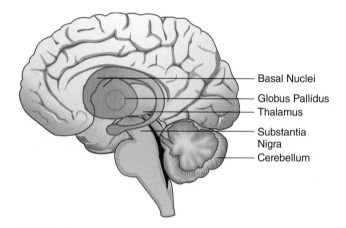

- Basal Nuclei
- Globus Pallidus
- Thalamus
- Substantia Nigra
- Cerebellum

FIGURE 1-14 **Basal nuclei (ganglia) and related structures.**

are the (1) caudate nucleus, (2) putamen, and (3) amygdala. The amygdala, as discussed earlier, is part of the limbic system and has little functional relationship with the remainder of the basal nuclei.

The remaining parts of the basal nuclei play a key role in generating complex motor programs for the body. In humans, the initial gross motor program developed in the basal nuclei must be fine-tuned by the motor areas of the cortex with which the basal nuclei communicate. Nerve fibers also connect the basal nuclei with the thalamus, subthalamus, and the substantia nigra in the midbrain in order to have highly coordinated motor function.

Parkinson's disease is a neurological disorder that is characterized by tremor, rigidity and akinesia. It is due to the degeneration, within the substantia nigra, of dopamine-producing cell bodies that have fibers that terminate in the basal nuclei. Damage to this pathway interferes with fine-tuned motor function needed for most common motor functions. A Parkinson-like syndrome (iatrogenic Parkinsonism) can also be caused by certain antipsychotic drugs that nonselectively block dopamine (DA) receptors throughout the brain.

NEUROPHYSIOLOGY OVERVIEW

There are two cardinal cell types in the nervous system: neurons and neuroglia. The neuron is the cell type that transmits or conducts signals within the nervous system. There are approximately 100 billion neurons in the human nervous system. The primary role of glial cells (known as Schwann cells in the peripheral nervous system) is to both support and insulate neurons, allowing for rapid, efficient communication and preventing electrical signals from spreading to areas where they shouldn't go.

The key components of a neuron (Figure 1-15) are:

- *Cell body.* It contains the neuron's nucleus and ribosomes, with the genetic information and tools necessary to make proteins.
- *Dendrites.* These branched outgrowths (may number in the thousands) from the cell body receive input from other neurons.
- *Axon.* This carries information from cell body to target. Collaterals may come off the axon to spread signals to larger areas.
- *Axon terminal.* Located at the end of the axon or collateral, it is the point from which neurotransmitters are released to act on a second neuron or a tissue.

INFORMATION EXCHANGE

In the nervous system, information is moved within the neuron from one end to the other (dendrites → cell body → axon) electrically, and between cells information is transferred chemically, using neurotransmitters to bridge the gap between one cell and the next.

Because of differences in (1) electric charge and (2) concentration of key ions (primarily, sodium and potassium [Na^+, and K^+], the interior of neurons has a relatively negative charge (−70 mV) compared to its surroundings (Figure 1-16). This charge difference is known as the cell's resting membrane potential. Any change in a cell's membrane potential (from −70 mV) produces electrical signals that are mediated by the movement of Na^+, and K^+ ions into and out of the neuron.

The change in membrane potential is cumulative and many signals may arrive simultaneously or sequentially from

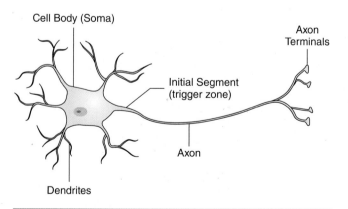

Cell Body (Soma)

Axon Terminals

Initial Segment (trigger zone)

Axon

Dendrites

FIGURE 1-15 **The key structures that make up a neuron are the dendrites, cell body, axon, and axon terminals.**

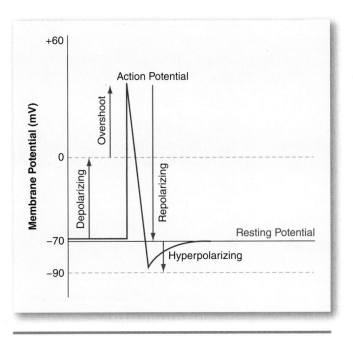

FIGURE 1-16 **During an action potential, as sodium enters the neuron, the interior of the cell becomes less negative (depolarization), and for a brief time the inside becomes positively charged. As potassium exits the cell, the membrane potential returns to resting level (repolarization) and the process is ready to begin anew.**

one neuron or from many neurons (up to several thousand). If the cumulative effect of this change in membrane potential is sufficient (i.e., reaches the threshold potential ~15 mV less negative than the resting membrane potential), it can trigger a powerful electrical signal, an action potential (AP), in the neuron. This occurs due to a massive influx of Na^+ (resulting from the opening of a specific sodium channel), and the neuron rapidly depolarizes (the electrical charge inside of the cell suddenly become positive relative to the outside of the cell). In just a tiny fraction of a second, a "gate" closes the Na^+ channel, K^+ channels open (K^+ flows out of cell), and the cell repolarizes. Finally, a specialized pump mechanism exchanges the Na^+ that was pumped in with the K^+ that was pumped out, allowing the cell to return to its resting membrane potential of −70 mV. This process then repeats itself again and again down the length of the neuron until the signal reaches the axon terminal. The number of APs moving through a given pathway in a given time (rate of transmission) determines the intensity of the stimulus (e.g., whisper vs. loud noise, touch vs. pinch).

Unfortunately, electrical signals cannot leap across the synaptic cleft, a minute gap (10 to 20 billionths of a meter) between neurons. Bridging that gap—to further pass information into, out of, or within the nervous system—requires a chemical molecule known as a neurotransmitter.

When an AP reaches the axon terminal, it triggers a process that encourages calcium (Ca^{++}) ions to enter the terminal. Most neurotransmitters are stored within synaptic vesicles, small storage sacs, in the terminals. The rise in intracellular Ca^{++} concentration in the axon terminal begins an elegantly choreographed performance in which the storage vesicles

belly up to and fuse with the cell membrane, releasing their contents into the synaptic cleft.

Across the synaptic cleft, on dendrites (or cell bodies) of the next neuron, are receptors for specific neurotransmitters. Depending on the neurotransmitter, binding with the receptor can depolarize the cell (membrane potential going from −70 mV to −65 mV, for example) or hyperpolarize the cell (−70 mV to −75 mV). Depolarization makes it easier to reach the threshold potential for the cell to generate an AP, whereas hyperpolarization makes it more difficult. A neuron may have thousands of synapses and the effect (AP or no AP) depends on the balance of excitatory (depolarizing) or inhibitory (hyperpolarizing) incoming signals received.

Physiologically, excitatory neurotransmitters generally open Na^+ channels (moving the membrane potential closer to the threshold potential). They may also slow conduction through K^+ or chloride (Cl^-) channels. Inhibitory neurotransmitters open K^+ channels (K^+ moves out) or increase Cl^- conductance (Cl^- moves in).

RECEPTORS

The concept of receptors for neurotransmitters dates back to the late nineteenth and early twentieth centuries. Based on several years of seemingly simple but elegant experiments by the renowned European physiologists Claude Bernard, J. N. Langley, T. R. Elliott, Otto Loewi, and Henry Dale, researchers concluded that motor neurons released a specialized chemical (acetylcholine), which caused muscles to twitch by combining with a mysterious receptive substance imbedded in the surface of the muscle tissue, and that this interaction began a series of unknown cellular changes that somehow caused the muscle to contract.

It is known that within the nervous system there may be as many as 50 to 100 neurotransmitters with a wide range of chemical compositions (Snyder & Ferris, 2000). More is also now known about receptors and what happens after a neurotransmitter binds to its receptor.

Starting at the receptor, there are two basic categories of receptor proteins: ionotropic (ligand-gated channels) and metabotropic (G-protein coupled). When a neurotransmitter (or drug) binds to an ionotropic receptor, it causes membrane ion channels to rapidly open or close, allowing the cell to very rapidly depolarize or hyperpolarize. When neurotransmitters bind to metabotropic receptors, a complex and coordinated cascade of intracellular changes takes place. These changes may cause channels to open or close, or other intracellular events may take place (e.g., enzyme activation or inhibition). These changes take place more slowly than ionotropic receptor events, but because of the additional steps, this pathway allows for amplification and modulation of signal, and for longer-lasting events. Ionotropic mechanisms are great for passing on discrete bits of information in a small cluster of cells whereas metabotropic mechanisms are more efficient when it is necessary to disseminate or modulate information over large and diffuse areas of the brain (Widmaier et al., 2008).

In the 1950s and 1960s, scientists identified a handful of brain neurotransmitters (norepinephrine, epinephrine, dopamine, and serotonin), each of which could act on receptors that often existed in multiple forms, or subtypes. For example, norepinephrine acts on alpha-1, alpha-2, beta-1, and beta-2 receptors, to affect different nervous system functions.

However, just when researchers were getting a handle on this small-scale elite group of neurotransmitters, their receptors, and the role they play in normal brain function and in mental illness, a host of new neurotransmitters was identified. These included the excitatory and inhibitory amino acids glutamate (GLU) and gamma-aminobutyric acid (GABA), respectively. In addition, dozens of peptides and a gas (nitric oxide, NO) are now recognized as neurotransmitters in the brain (Boehning & Snyder, 2003).

NEUROTRANSMITTERS

This section examines specific neurotransmitters that are critical to normal brain function and their possible role in mental illness. Many of these neurotransmitters are also discussed in later chapters since they are targets for the action of psychotropic drugs.

ACETYLCHOLINE (ACh)

The first neurotransmitter ever identified was acetylcholine (ACh). In 1914, while an undergraduate student at Trinity College, in London, the British physiologist Henry Dale discovered a chemical produced in nature by rye fungus that had actions on animal organs similar to those produced by nerves. He named the chemical acetylcholine. Seven years later, in 1921, the German-American pharmacologist Otto Loewi discovered an unidentified chemical released by nerves innervating the (frog) heart, which he named *vagusstoff*, or "vagus substance." When Dale heard of Loewi's fantastic discovery, he thought Loewi's vagusstoff might be identical to the chemical he had discovered earlier, ACh. He was right. Together, Loewi and Dale shared the 1936 Nobel Prize for Physiology or Medicine "for their discoveries relating to chemical transmission of nerve impulses." The first neurotransmitter, acetylcholine, had two fathers, a pair of the finest minds of their generation.

Acetylcholine is a key neurotransmitter in both the peripheral and central nervous system. In most instances ACh is an excitatory neurotransmitter, although peripherally vagal innervation of the heart is inhibitory. It has two basic subtypes of receptors: nicotinic (ionotropic—skeletal muscle contraction) and muscarinic (metabotropic—smooth muscle and glands).

ACh is secreted by neurons in several regions of the brain (Figure 1-17), including multiple areas of the cerebral cortex and in the basal nuclei. However, the nucleus basalis of Meynert (NBM) is the brain center where most cholinergic neuron cell bodies that project throughout the brain originate. This is a small area in the substantia innominata, a layer of cells in the forebrain just below the anterior thalamus.

Degeneration of neurons in NBM is where the earliest damage to the brain is thought to occur in Alzheimer's disease. Over time, the damage becomes more widespread and additional areas of the brain innervated by the NBM (e.g., hippocampus and amygdala) begin to die off. As the disease continues to progress, diffuse damage to the neocortex occurs. Drugs that elevate brain acetylcholine levels are used, with limited effectiveness, in patients with Alzheimer's disease.

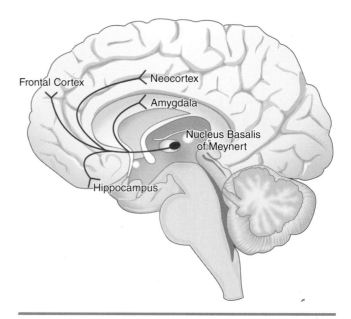

FIGURE 1-17 **Primary pathways from the nucleus basalis of Meynert that release acetylcholine in the frontal cortex, neocortex, amygdala, and hippocampus.**

The presence of nicotinic receptors for acetylcholine in reward pathways in the brain is believed to underlie the addictive properties of tobacco (nicotine)[6]. In 2006, the FDA approved varenicline (Chantix), a drug that interferes with nicotine's (rewarding) action in the brain, for smoking cessation (Potts & Garwood, 2007).

BIOGENIC AMINES: NOREPINEPHRINE (NE), DOPAMINE (DA), AND SEROTONIN (5-HT)

Biogenic amines are small neurotransmitter molecules synthesized from amino acids. In the peripheral nervous system the main biogenic amine neurotransmitters are norepinephrine and epinephrine. In the brain the key biogenic amine neurotransmitters are norepinephrine, dopamine, and serotonin.

Norepinephrine (NE) is released by neurons in the brain whose cell bodies are found primarily in the brainstem and hypothalamus (Figure 1-18). The locus ceruleus is a key source for cell bodies in the pons that innervate several areas of the brain. Projections from the LC go to the frontal cortex where NE may control, or at least influence, mood, attention, concentration, working memory, and speed of information processing. Projections to the limbic system may mediate emotions, feelings of energy, fatigue, psychomotor agitation, or psychomotor retardation.

After NE is released by nerve endings and interacts with postsynaptic receptors, its action is terminated by one of three

---

[6]Nicotine, despite being addictive, is not that harmful to human tissue. However, the major vehicle for getting nicotine into the body, cigarettes, contains a variety of carcinogenic substances, which enter the body as well. Nicotine thus drives people to engage in self-injurious behaviors, a classic sign of an addictive drug.

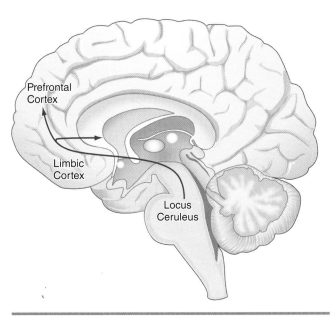

FIGURE 1-18 Primary norepinephrine pathways from the locus ceruleus to the prefrontal cortex and the limbic system.

processes, the most important of which is reuptake by the neuron that released the NE; it is taken back up into storage vesicles and later reused (Figure 1-19).

In these pathways, along with dopamine, NE may play a key role in the development of attention deficit hyperactivity disorder (ADHD) and likely contributes to some of the behavioral effects that occur when stimulants, such as amphetamines and cocaine, are abused. It also may serve an important role in depression, or at least in the treatment of depression.

Among the earliest and most effective drugs used to treat depression are two classes of drugs that raise synaptic NE (and serotonin or 5-HT) levels in the brain. One class of drugs, the tricyclic antidepressants (TCAs) interfere with the neuronal reuptake process, which raises synaptic NE and 5-HT levels, allowing more of these neurotransmitters to interact with receptors for longer periods. The second class of drugs, the monoamine oxidase inhibitors (MAOIs) have a similar effect on synaptic NE levels but do so by interfering with the breakdown of NE within the nerve terminal, so that more NE is released with each AP reaching the terminal.

It is known that the beneficial effects of these drugs on depression is very complex and that these actions may be just the beginning of a cascade of neurochemical effects that take up to several weeks to complete (see Chapter 2).

Dopamine (DA), while primarily a precursor molecule for the synthesis of epinephrine and norepinephrine in the peripheral (autonomic) nervous system, is an important neurotransmitter in the brain. There are several key DA pathways in the brain (Figure 1-20) involved in hormonal activities (tuberoinfundibular), motor function (nigrostriatal), and reward pathways (mesolimbic and mesocortical). Disturbances in both the mesolimbic and mesocortical pathways are believed to play a role in schizophrenia and other psychoses.

Beginning in the 1960s, until at least the mid-1980s, all drugs used to treat schizophrenia blocked DA receptors in the brain. These drugs specifically blocked the D_2 subtype of the receptor, supporting the basic theory that in schizophrenia

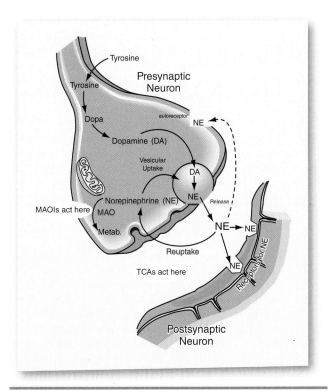

FIGURE 1-19 Presynaptic and postsynaptic neurons, showing the synthesis of norepinephrine (NE), its release, action on pre- and postsynaptic receptors, as well as reuptake of NE. Also shown are the sites of action for MAO inhibitors and tricyclic antidepressants.

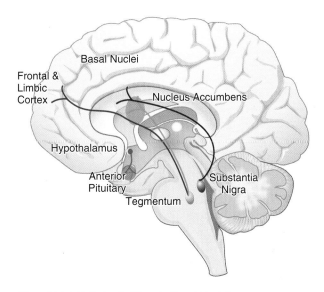

Nigrostriatal (Substantia Nigra to Basal Nuclei)
Mesolimbic (Ventral Tegmentum to Nucleus Accumbens)
Mesocortical (Ventral Tegmentum to Frontal and Limbic Cortex)
Tuberoinfundibular (Hypothalamus to Anterior Pituitary)

FIGURE 1-20 Shown are the four primary dopamine pathways in the brain.

patients had excessive DA activity in certain parts of the brain and this was the neurochemical basis for this disorder (Stahl, 2008). DA-receptor-blocking drugs, beginning with chlorpromazine (Thorazine), profoundly helped these patients function in society. However, they also produced a host of neurological (and other) adverse effects because they blocked DA receptors throughout the brain, not just those in areas "causing" the schizophrenia.

Newer drugs for schizophrenia, beginning with the use of clozapine (Clozaril), not only affect DA receptors but also block certain serotonin receptors (5-HT$_{2A}$). The overall effect is a greater range of effectiveness with fewer adverse effects. The role of DA and serotonin in psychoses is addressed in Chapter 4.

Both the mesolimbic and the mesocortical pathways play critical roles in the brain's reward and pleasure centers. Drugs that elevate DA levels in these areas of the brain have a high potential for abuse. These include cocaine and amphetamines, which directly elevate DA levels, and opioids and alcohol, which may indirectly elevate DA levels.

Serotonin (5-hydroxytryptamine or 5-HT) is another key biogenic amine neurotransmitter in both the central and peripheral nervous system and is also found in other parts of the body (e.g., platelets, immune system, and digestive tract). In fact, only 1% to 2% of the body's serotonin is found in the brain.

In 1948, researchers at the Cleveland Clinic discovered a chemical vasoconstrictor released by clots into serum (Sneader, 2005). They named it serotonin (*sero* . . . —serum agent; . . . *tonin*—affecting vascular tone). Serotonin was soon chemically identified as 5-hydroxytryptamine and found to have a broad range of physiological roles, including that of a neurotransmitter in the nervous system. Most serotonergic neurons in the CNS are located in the raphe nucleus of the brainstem (Figure 1-21).

There are at least seven major subtypes of serotonin receptors, many of which have their own subtypes (e.g.,

5-HT$_{1A}$, 5-HT$_{2A}$, 5-HT$_{2C}$ . . .). This neurotransmitter is involved in regulating a wide range of neurophysiological functions including mood, sleep, appetite, nausea, body temperature, blood pressure, and pain perception. Serotonin appears to be involved in clinical conditions such as depression (see Chapter 2), schizophrenia (see Chapter 4), anxiety (see Chapter 6), migraine, and irritable bowel syndrome (not covered in this text).

Drugs, such as fluoxetine (Prozac), that inhibit neuronal reuptake of serotonin are used to treat depression. Several second-generation antipsychotic drugs, including risperidone (Risperidal), block 5-HT$_{2A}$ receptors. Buspirone (BuSpar), a 5-HT$_{1A}$ agonist, is used for anxiety. Other 5-HT agonists are used to treat migraine and still others are used for irritable bowel syndrome. The 5-HT antagonists are commonly used to treat or prevent nausea, particularly when it is caused by chemotherapy.

AMINO ACID NEUROTRANSMITTERS ✓

Glutamate (GLU) is the principal and most common excitatory neurotransmitter in the nervous system. It is found in more than 50% of all synapses in the CNS (Snyder & Ferris, 2000). There are several GLU receptors, the two most important of which (discovered so far) are the AMPA and the NMDA subtypes. On cells where both of these receptors are co-localized, they work cooperatively to produce long-term potentiation, a key process involved in learning and memory.

However, NMDA receptors for GLU also seem to play an insidious role in a process known as excitotoxicity. When GLU-containing brain cells (of which there are many) die or are injured, massive amounts of GLU may be released. This very high GLU concentration can overstimulate nearby neurons (by raising intracellular calcium levels), causing them to die. If these cells also contain GLU, the damage can spread rapidly. Several clinical studies indicate that administering NMDA antagonists can minimize the spread of cell death following injury (a stroke), suggesting a vital role for the NMDA-receptor subtype in this dying-off process (Lees, 1997). Numerous studies are being carried out to explore the potential benefit of NMDA antagonists in treating strokes; traumatic brain injuries; epilepsy; Alzheimer's; Parkinson's and Huntington's diseases; and mood disorders. However, despite the apparent positive clinical potential of this class of drugs, they may also have a dark side. Several studies have found that NMDA antagonists may be neurotoxic (Davis et al., 2000; Olney, Labruyere, & Price, 1989).

GABA (gamma amino butyric acid) is the principal inhibitory transmitter in the brain (Figure 1-22) (Meldrum, 1982). It is released primarily by interneurons. The two main subtypes of GABA receptors are GABA$_A$ and GABA$_B$.

GABA hyperpolarizes neurons by opening chloride channels, so that a stronger signal is required to produce an action potential. Most drugs that act via the neurotransmitter GABA (e.g., benzodiazepines and barbiturates), do not bind to the GABA binding site. In fact this receptor is actually a complex with multiple binding sites for other chemicals/drugs (Figure 1-22).

When benzodiazepines and barbiturates attach to their binding sites, chloride rushes into the cell much more rapidly

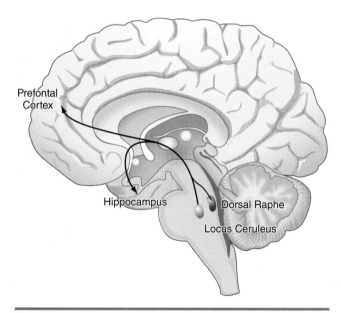

FIGURE 1-21 Shown are major 5-HT pathways in the brain and originating in the dorsal raphe nucleus.

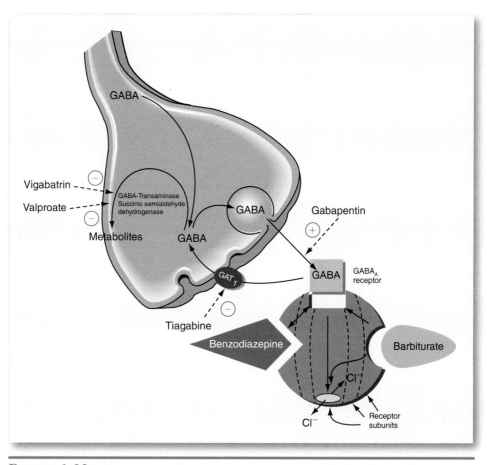

FIGURE 1-22 GABA-receptor binding complex. Receptor has binding site for GABA, which opens chloride channels. On the receptor complex are secondary binding sites for benzodiazepines and barbiturates.

than when GABA attaches to its binding site in their absence (Charney, Mihic, & Harris, 2006; McNamara, 2006). The extra Cl^- entering the cell makes it harder to trigger an action potential. By definition, therefore, these drugs are CNS depressants.

THE COMPLEX BRAIN

Information travels unidirectionally in the nervous system. Action potentials travel down an axon from the soma to the axon terminal. This triggers the release of a neurotransmitter to act on a specific dendritic receptors for that neurotransmitter on the target cell, and this process continues for as long as necessary. This dogma of neurotransmission, accepted for over a century, is not as neat and tidy as it seems. In fact nothing is simple or straightforward in the brain.

According to *Dorland's Electronic Medical Dictionary* (Dorland, 2009), a neurotransmitter is "a substance . . . that is released from the axon terminal of a presynaptic neuron on excitation, and that travels across the synaptic cleft to either excite or inhibit the target cell." This is not always a just a two-player (NT and receptor) game and other players in this process include neuromodulators. Neuromodulators are chemicals released by a neuron at a synapse that conveys information by either enhancing or dampening the activities at adjacent or distant neurons (Boehning & Snyder, 2003). This sounds like the description of a neurotransmitter, but not quite.

Norepinephrine, dopamine, serotonin, and acetylcholine are classic neurotransmitters and their very existence, release, site of action, and destruction have been used to define a chemical messenger as a neurotransmitter. Peptides released by neurons act much more slowly than classic neurotransmitters, have receptors that may not be adjacent to their release site, and may influence the effect of a neurotransmitter on its receptor. As such, they are often referred to as neuromodulators.

The role of the neuromodulator is similar to that of the fine-tuner that once worked with the old black-and-white televisions. These televisions came equipped with both a tuner and a fine-tuner. The tuner allowed the viewer to choose one of the stations that was available, but the signal had to be adjusted with the fine-tuner to bring it in clearly. In neurotransmission parlance, a neuromodulator is to the neurotransmitter what the fine-tuner was to the old television tuner; it helps bring the signal into clear focus.

NEUROPEPTIDE MESSENGERS

Neuropeptides are sequences of two or more amino acids that have neurotransmitter-like activity in the nervous system. Over 85 neuropeptides have been identified although their physiological roles in neurotransmission are mostly a mystery (Boehning & Snyder, 2003; Snyder & Ferris, 2000). Examples of neuropeptides include: angiotensin, bradykinin, calcitonin, cholecystokinin, delta sleep-inducing peptide, gastric inhibitory polypeptide, melanocyte-stimulating hormone, neuropeptide Y, neurotensin, pancreatic polypeptide, secretin, vasoactive intestinal peptide, vasopressin, tachykinins, calcitonin gene-related peptide, opioid peptides, gastrin-releasing peptide, substance P, and thyrotropin-releasing hormone. Most of these neuropeptides have hormonal action outside of the nervous system.

MULTIPLE RELEASES

Certain neurons produce and release a small molecule neurotransmitter and one or more neuropeptides. Within the neurons these chemicals are contained in the same or in different types of vesicles and their release may be differentially regulated. Table 1-2 presents some examples of this. The role of neuropeptide neuromodulators in specific disease states or those associated with psychotropic drug actions are discussed later.

NEURONAL MESSENGERS

In the last two decades, certain gases are now accepted as neuronal chemical messengers (neurotransmitters or neuromodulators) in humans (Boehning & Snyder, 2003). These gases include nitric oxide (NO, the same gas that comes out of a car's exhaust pipe), carbon monoxide (CO, the molecule that gives people rosy red cheeks while it kills them), and hydrogen sulfide (H_2S, the chemical that gives rotten eggs their potent smell). None of these gases, however, are found in neuronal vesicles nor do they bind to receptors. In fact, hydrogen sulfide is not even made in neurons (it is produced in astrocytes, a type of glial cell). In many ways these chemicals defy the very definition of neurotransmitter. Yet, they clearly convey neuronal information. Furthermore, they convey that information in reverse; that is, from the dendrite of the postsynaptic cell to the axon terminal of the presynaptic cell. They are, in other words, retrograde transmitters.

✓ RETROGRADE MESSENGERS

An example of the retrograde feedback process can be seen in the hippocampus through the action of NO. In the hippocampus, GLU acts on NMDA (and AMPA) receptors to open calcium channels. The incoming calcium then initiates a process that elevates postsynaptic NO levels. NO diffuses out of the cell into the interstitial space (synaptic cleft) and then is taken up by presynaptic GLU-releasing cells where it facilitates the release of more GLU. NO thus acts as a retrograde messenger and this feedback process is a key element of long-term potentiation (LTP), believed to be the basis of learning and memory.

NO plays a wide number of roles in the central and peripheral nervous system and in vasculature. It is known to affect learning, development, drug tolerance, sensory and motor modulation, bronchial function, and penile erection (basis for sildenafil [Viagra] action). The roles of CO and H_2S are not discussed in this text.

This tidy categorical distinction between neurotransmitter and neuromodulator may be somewhat arbitrary and not so clear-cut after all. For example, compare and contrast the neurotransmitters GLU and NE (Figure 1-23). GLU is a ubiquitous, fast-acting (few milliseconds) neurotransmitter in the brain that acts locally and rapidly, and transmits discrete bits of information over very short distances. NE, on the other hand, is contained in clumps of neurons in well-defined areas of the brain, acts relatively slowly (100 milliseconds or

TABLE 1-2 Neurotransmitters and Neuropeptide Co-Transmitters

NEUROTRANSMITTER	NEUROPEPTIDE CO-TRANSMITTER
Norepinephrine (neurons of the A2 cell group in the nucleus of the solitary tract)	Galanin Enkephalin Neuropeptide Y
GABA	Somatostatin (in the hippocampus) Cholecystokinin Neuropeptide Y (in the arcuate nucleus)
Acetylcholine	VIP Substance P
Dopamine	Cholecystokinin Neurotensin
Epinephrine	Neuropeptide Y Neurotensin
Serotonin (5-HT)	Substance P TRH Enkephalin

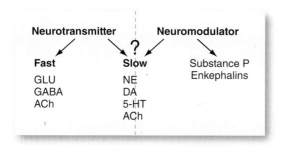

FIGURE 1-23 Classification of chemicals that act in the brain as fast or slow neurotransmitters or as neuromodulators.

longer), and influences far-flung, remote regions of the brain. Because of the sluggish response times, slow neurotransmitters have greater opportunity to interact with and modulate their targets. Within this context, Mendoza and Foundas, in their text *Clinical Neuroanatomy: A Neurobehavioral Approach* (2007), refer to slow neurotransmitters as neuromodulators. To a certain degree it is a matter of semantics as to whether NE (or DA or 5-HT) is called a slow neurotransmitter or a neuromodulator. Acetylcholine, in different parts of the nervous system, is both a fast and a slow neurotransmitter. In the brain and at skeletal muscle it acts as a fast transmitter, but in the periphery, at exocrine glands and smooth muscles, it acts as a slow neurotransmitter. For clarity, this text refers to the small molecule transmitters (slow or fast) as neurotransmitters and neuropeptides as neuromodulators. Classification of the gases is not addressed.

Unusual Messengers

D-serine is another one of those chemicals produced in the brain that affects neurotransmission but does not fit the classic definition of a neurotransmitter or neuromodulator, primarily because it is released not by neurons but by glial cells (Boehning & Snyder, 2003). Upon release it binds to postsynaptic NMDA receptors for the neurotransmitter GLU. It appears that NMDA receptors are unique in that they require two different neurotransmitters (GLU and D-serine) to bind at the same time before Ca^{+2} channels are opened.

Another unusual group of messengers is the endocannabinoids. The name *cannabinoid* should look familiar since Δ^9-tetrahydrocannabinol is the active ingredient in marijuana. The endocannabinoids (N-arachidonoyl ethanolamine and 1-arachidonoylglycerol) are endogenous cannabinoid neuronal messengers found in mammalian organs, especially in the brain (Akopian, Ruparel, Jeske, Patwardhan, & Hargreaves, 2009). The endocannabinoids appear to be important modulators for such diverse physiological processes as learning, memory, appetite control, and reward, as well as in certain pathological processes such as pain, anxiety, and mood disorders. These actions are consistent with the "clinical" (mis) use of cannabinoids. These cannabinoids are produced in the brain on an as-needed basis (i.e., they are not stored), released by postsynaptic neurons, and act on specific presynaptic cannabinoid receptors (CB1) on both GLU and GABA neurons. In this manner, the cannabinoids are retrograde signal molecules that provide feedback and modulate the release of additional neurotransmitter.

NEUROTROPHINS

Neurotrophic factors or neurotrophins are growth factors that are capable of signaling neurons to survive, differentiate, or grow. They are critical in brain development as neurons form. They also play a role later in life regulating apoptosis (programmed cell death), neurogenesis, and neuroplasticity. One neurotrophin in particular, brain-derived neurotrophic factor (BDNF) is addressed in Chapter 2, since it may play a key role in the causation and the possible treatment of several brain disorders.

INFORMATION GATHERING

There are atleast four ways that are used to gather information about the brain. The oldest method involves observing changes in behavior following known brain injuries (trauma, tumors, etc.). If damage to a known area of the brain affects a certain behavior, it is not unreasonable to conclude that the damaged area of the brain regulates that behavior. Perhaps the most famous example of this was the 25-year-old Vermont railroad foreman Phineas Gage who, in 1848, suffered an unfortunate accident. Mr. Gage was tamping down a blasting charge when the powder exploded prematurely and the 3½-foot-long by 1¼-inch-diameter iron rod he was using was driven up through and out of his head with enough force to carry it 80 feet away. An estimate of its path is shown in Figure 1-24 from the paper written in 1868 by John Harlow, the physician who treated Mr. Gage for his injury. It is agreed that, at a minimum, Gage's left frontal lobe, and possibly both frontal lobes, suffered serious damage from the injury, which he not only survived but walked away from.

In terms of the change in Mr. Gage's personality after the accident, Harlow notes in his report (1868), "He is fitful, irreverent, indulging at times in the grossest profanity (which

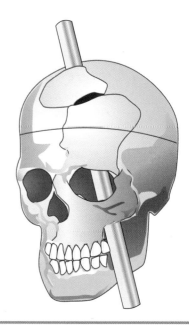

FIGURE 1-24 An estimate of the path of the iron rod through the skull of Phineas Gage (From the paper written in 1868 by John Harlow).

was not previously his custom), manifesting but little deference for his fellows, impatient of restraint or advice when it conflicts with his desires, at times pertinaciously obstinate, yet capricious and vacillating. . . . In this regard his mind was radically changed, so decidedly that his friends and acquaintances said he was 'no longer Gage.'"

A second source of information comes from simply observing and recording the behavior of other mammals. As brain surgery has become more common, it provides a third way to understand the workings of the brain. Because the human brain doesn't have much in the way of sensory neurons (no pain), brain surgery is often performed while the patient is conscious. As probes are pushed and prodded into different areas of the brain, patients can report what they are experiencing.

One of the newest techniques for understanding how the brain works is known as functional magnetic resonance imaging, or fMRI. This form of brain imaging registers blood flow to various areas of the brain. The more active the area, the higher its blood flow and the "brighter" it shows up on an fMRI scan.

Whereas traditional magnetic resonance imaging (MRI) examines anatomy, fMRI opens a window to study metabolic activity of the brain, in real-time, when an event is occurring. The fMRI, in other words, is a way of correlating function (physiology) with form (anatomy). The potential of this powerful new tool and others (single photon emission computerized tomography—SPECT, positron emission tomography—PET, magneto-encephalography—MEG, and magnetic resonance spectroscopy—MRS) can only be imagined. It is important to evaluate how best to use these new tools and to note their potential limitations in order to prevent misuse or overuse.

REVIEW QUESTIONS

1. What term best describes the normal functions of the human nervous system?
   a. Neurotransmitter
   b. Neuroanatomy
   c. Neuropeptide
   d. Neurophysiology

2. Beginning above the spinal cord, what is the lowest section of the brain?
   a. Cerebellum
   b. Hypothalamus
   c. Cerebrum
   d. Brainstem

For the next 4 questions, pick the best answer from below. Each answer may be used once, more than once, or not at all.
   a. Substantia nigra – *dopamine degeneration*
   b. Raphe nuclei – *secrete 5-HT*
   c. Hypothalamus – *hormones*
   d. Hippocampus – *memory*

3. An area of the brain that plays a key role in memory is the _____ __.

4. Dopamine (DA)-producing cell bodies originating in the ___*pleasure*___ innervate the basal nuclei and help coordinate movement and muscle tone. Degeneration of this region is believed to be the root cause of Parkinsonism.

5. Most serotonergic neurons in the CNS are located in the _____ of the brainstem.

6. The region of the brain in which the nervous system and the endocrine system intersect and communicate with each other is the _____.

7. What is the primary advantage of all the folding of brain tissue in the cerebrum?
   a. Shorter distances between neurons for rapid communication.
   b. Increased surface area in a limited space.
   c. Both *a* and *b* are correct.
   d. Neither *a* or *b* are correct.

8. Which of the following statements regarding acetylcholine is false?
   a. It was the first neurotransmitter identified, and it was initially named vagusstoff.
   b. It is a neurotransmitter in both the central and peripheral nervous system.
   c. It is the most common excitatory neurotransmitter in the nervous system.
   d. The loss of cholinergic neurons in the brain appears to be the pathophysiological basis of Alzheimer's disease.

9. Which neurotransmitter is most involved in reward pathways in the brain?
   a. Acetylcholine
   b. GABA
   c. Nitric oxide
   d. Dopamine

10. The active ingredient in marijuana, Δ^9-tetrahydrocannabinol, is believed to act at receptors for endogenous cannabinoid neuronal messengers.
   a. True
   b. False

REFERENCES

Akopian, A. N., Ruparel, N. B., Jeske, N. A., Patwardhan, A., & Hargreaves, K. M. (2009). Role of ionotropic cannabinoid receptors in peripheral antinociception and antihyperalgesia. *Trends in Pharmacological Sciences, 30*(2), 79–84.

Boehning, D., & Snyder, S. H. (2003). Novel neural modulators. *Annual Review of Neuroscience, 26*, 105–131.

Charney, D. S., Mihic, S. J., & Harris, R. A. (2006). Hypnotics and sedatives. In L. L. Brunton, J. S. Lazo, & K. L. Parker (Eds.), *Goodman & Gilman's the pharmacological basis of therapeutics* (11th ed.). New York: McGraw-Hill.

Davis, S. M., Lees, K. R., Albers, G. W., Diener, H. C., Markabi, S., Karlsson, G., et al. (2000). Selfotel in acute ischemic stroke: Possible neurotoxic effects of an NMDA antagonist. *Stroke; a Journal of Cerebral Circulation, 31*(2), 347–354.

DiPiro, J. T., Talbert, R. L., Yee, G. C., Matzke, G. R., & Wells, B. G. (2008). *Pharmacotherapy: A pathophysiologic approach.* New York: McGraw-Hill Medical.

Dorland. *Dorland's electronic medical dictionary,* 31st ed. Retrieved 5/27/2009, 2009, from http://www.dorlands.com/wsearch.jsp

Harlow, J. M. (1868). Recovery from the passage of an iron bar through the head. *Publications of Massachusetts Medical Society, 2,* 327–347.

Hashimoto, T., Tayama, M., Murakawa, K., Yoshimoto, T., Miyazaki, M., Harada, M., et al. (1995). Development of the brainstem and cerebellum in autistic patients. *Journal of Autism and Developmental Disorders, 25*(1), 1–18.

Lees, K. R. (1997). Cerestat and other NMDA antagonists in ischemic stroke. *Neurology, 49*(5 Suppl 4), S66–S69.

Linden, D. J. (2008). *The accidental mind: How brain evolution has given us love, memory, dreams, and god* (1st ed.). Cambridge, MA: The Belknap Press.

McNamara, J. O. (2006). Pharmacotherapy of the epilepsies. In L. L. Brunton, J. S. Lazo & K. L. Parker (Eds.), *Goodman & Gilman's the pharmacological basis of therapeutics* (11th ed.). New York: McGraw-Hill.

Meldrum, B. (1982). Pharmacology of GABA. *Clinical Neuropharmacology, 5*(3), 293–316.

Mendoza, J., & Foundas, A. L. (2007). *Clinical neuroanatomy: A neurobehavioral approach* (1st ed.). New York: Springer.

Naqvi, N. H., Rudrauf, D., Damasio, H., & Bechara, A. (2007). Damage to the insula disrupts addiction to cigarette smoking. *Science, 315*(5811), 531–534.

Olney, J. W., Labruyere, J., & Price, M. T. (1989). Pathological changes induced in cerebrocortical neurons by phencyclidine and related drugs. *Science, 244*(4910), 1360–1362.

Oregon Public Broadcasting. *Rediscovering biology—online textbook: Unit 10 neurobiology.* Retrieved 5/26/2009, 2009, from http://www.learner.org/courses/biology/textbook/neuro/index.html

Potts, L. A., & Garwood, C. L. (2007). Varenicline: The newest agent for smoking cessation. *American Journal of Health-System Pharmacy, 64*(13), 1381–1384.

Sneader, W. (2005). *Drug discovery: A history* (1st ed.). Chichester: Wiley-Interscience.

Snyder, S. H., & Ferris, C. D. (2000). Novel neurotransmitters and their neuropsychiatric relevance. *American Journal of Psychiatry, 157*(11), 1738.

Society for Neuroscience. (2008). *Brain facts : A primer of the brain and nervous system.* Retrieved 5/26/2009, 2009, from http://www.sfn.org/skins/main/pdf/brainfacts/2008/brain_facts.pdf

Stahl, S. M. (2008). *Stahl's essential psychopharmacology: Neuroscientific basis and practical applications* (3rd ed.). New York: Cambridge University Press.

Widmaier, E. P., Vander, A. J., Raff, H., & Strang, K. T. (2006). *Vander's human physiology: the mechanisms of body function.* Boston: McGraw-Hill.

CHAPTER 2
Pharmacotherapy of Depression

"In addition to my other numerous acquaintances, I have one more intimate confidant. My depression is the most faithful mistress I have known—no wonder, then, that I return the love."

SØREN KIERKEGAARD

GETTING PERSONAL

I couldn't breathe.

Every morning was a struggle and I didn't want to get out of bed. I didn't want to eat and I wouldn't talk to anyone. My wife of almost 35 years died four months earlier from a recurrence of lung cancer after almost a year of remission. At first, I thought I was handling her death quite well. The first few weeks I was appropriately grief stricken and despondent, but I had to get back to living so I went to work and talked with friends and family about my/our loss. These were appropriate responses given what I had gone through.

What I did not seek, however, was grief counseling. Who needed it? I had gotten through the tough part already, hadn't I? Then, I didn't have to work for the summer and I had (way too much) time to think and reflect on my life and my loss. Within a month, I lost my appetite and when I ate my stomach got upset. I had difficulty sleeping and when I woke up early in the morning, I felt like I was having a panic attack. I could hardly breathe and I wasn't sure how I would get through the day. I stopped enjoying the company of others. I wanted to be alone and I stayed in bed all day reading spy novels. It was the only way I could distract myself. I tried straightening up my house, but every drawer I opened brought back wonderful memories and crushing waves of sadness, so I retreated to my book. I couldn't work on any of the summer projects I had planned without becoming overwhelmed and paralyzed.

After five weeks of feeling helpless and lost, I talked with a friend who happened to be a psychiatric nurse. Her immediate impression was that I was depressed. She urged me to consult my personal physician, who put me on an antidepressant.

It took about six weeks before I even approached feeling like my old self. After losing almost 20 pounds, I began to eat again, and I could wake up in the morning without feeling anxious. I began to talk to friends again without feeling like the biggest idiot in town, someone who no one wanted to be around. I got my "mojo" back. As I'm writing this, it's been about nine months since my wife died and I've been on an antidepressant for about five months. I'm not sure what would have happened if I hadn't been pushed to get help by family and friends and I'm glad I never got to find out.

Anonymous

DIAGNOSING DEPRESSION

According to the Diagnostic and Statistical Manual of Mental Disorders (DSM-IV-TR), a major depressive episode is defined as at least two weeks of depressed mood or loss of interest, accompanied by four or more of the following symptoms: change in appetite or weight, sleep disturbance, psychomotor agitation or slowing, fatigue or loss of energy, worthlessness or guilt, poor concentration or indecisiveness, and thoughts of suicide or death. Often people dealing with these symptoms will not use the word *depression*. Instead they may use words such as: *stressed out, unhappy, sad, melancholic, miserable, sorrowful, woeful, gloomy, despondent, in low spirits, having a heavy heart, in despair, desolate, hopeless, upset, tearful, in the dumps, having the doldrums, having the blues,* or *in a funk.* Yet, according to Rakel & Bope (2008), despite widespread inability to find the right words to describe the ailment, depression is the fourth most common complaint seen in a primary care setting. About one in every ten patients seen by a primary care provider has a major depressive disorder. In fact, according to the authors, 68% of patients who overuse medical care have, at some time in their lives, had a diagnosis of major depression. Although the presentation of depression may or may not include crying jags, it may include a dramatic increase in somatic complaints (Kroenke, 2003).

The topic of depression may be approached from many directions; this text focuses on the drugs or antidepressants used to treat the disorder. However, it is not possible to discuss antidepressants without mentioning the underlying illness. The advent of antidepressant drugs has helped researchers understand the neurochemical basis of depression, and without these drugs depression still might be viewed as a character flaw, rather than as a biological disorder related to neurochemicals in the brain.

Mood disorders can be unipolar or bipolar, as seen in Figure 2-1. Patients with unipolar depression may have a single major depressive episode in their lifetime or it may be a recurrent problem, separated by periods of euthymia or normal mood. Patients who have bipolar mood disorders (see Chapter 3) alternate between episodes of depression and mania, with each episode varying in duration. These episodes may be separated by periods of euthymia or they may cycle rapidly or even occur concurrently.

BATTLING DEPRESSION

It may be helpful for the clinician to think like a field general in the war against depression. The battlefield is the disease and the patient is a soldier under the clinician's care and supervision. Together the clinician and patient implement a battle plan using the most effective weapons available to defeat depression. While drugs are part of the clinician's treatment arsenal, they are not the only weapons available.

THE FOUR RS: RECOVERY, REMISSION, RESPONSE, AND RECURRENCE

Depression is a tough adversary and the clinician and patient must be prepared for a prolonged and perhaps lifelong war, which is fought one battle at a time. Depression (unipolar or bipolar) is often a recurring illness, with each occurrence representing a battle (Figure 2-2). The goal is to arm the patient, with powerful weapons (including drugs), to attain full recovery. Recovery is defined as having no signs of depression for over a year after the last battle or depressive episode. Until this point, if there is no evidence of depression, the patient is in remission.

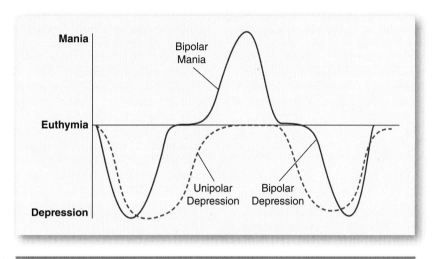

FIGURE 2-1 Time course of unipolar (dashed line) depression and bipolar mood disorder (solid line).

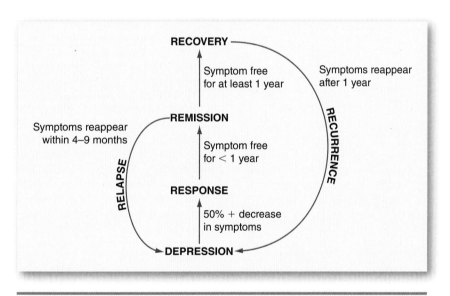

FIGURE 2-2 Stages in the recovery from depression, including the intermediary steps of response and remission as well as the loss of benefit (relapse and recurrence).

Sometimes, a drug does not completely defeat the symptoms, but it does significantly weaken the depression (at least a 50% decrease in symptoms). This is a positive response. Unfortunately, many clinicians are satisfied with a positive response and terminate drug treatment before true remission occurs. Too often, this leads to relapse (another battle or depressive episode within four to nine months of the previous battle) or recurrence (a depressive episode after one year of remission). It is important to set a goal of remission and recovery at the start of the first battle with depression, and not just accept a positive response as success. Each clinical failure makes it more likely that more battles will have to be fought in the future.

What is currently known about depression and the antidepressants? What causes this disease and how do the drugs used to treat it work? In order to gain an understanding of

depression it is necessary to see that these questions are interrelated; the current information available about one question helps to expand the knowledge about the other.

BIOLOGIC PSYCHIATRY

Tuberculosis is a respiratory disorder that has afflicted millions of people for centuries. The cure for the disease was time and isolation from other people to prevent its spread because there was no effective drug treatment for tuberculosis. However, in 1951 two physicians in a New York hospital discovered that isoniazid, a derivative of hydrazine (a propellant used by the Germans in World War II for the V2 rockets), effectively stopped tuberculosis (Healy, 1997; Selikoff & Robitzek, 1952). By chance, clinicians also observed that the mood of patients in tuberculosis sanatoriums improved with isoniazid or iproniazid. Actually, the mood of nontubercular depressed patients improved as well, and improved consistently, even when treated with a derivative of isoniazid that lacked antitubercular properties (isocarboxazid—Marplan). So, how do these drugs work to treat depression? To answer this question it is necessary to look at their neurochemical effects in the brain.

MONOAMINE OXIDASE INHIBITORS (MAOIs)

The first antidepressants shared one attribute. They all inhibited neuronal monoamine oxidase (MAO), an enzyme that breaks down monoamine neurotransmitters such as norepinephrine (NE) and serotonin (5-HT). When MAO is inhibited, less NE or 5-HT is metabolized in the neuron and more of these transmitters are available to be released and to act on other neurons in the nervous system. Figure 2-3 shows the synthesis, release, metabolism, and reuptake of NE. Essentially the same events occur in neurons that release 5-HT.

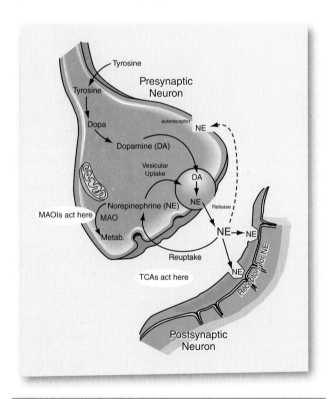

FIGURE 2-3 Synthesis, release, reuptake, and metabolism of norepinephrine (NE). Tyrosine, an amino acid, is taken up by neurons and is sequentially metabolized to DOPA, then dopamine (DA). The DA is taken up into vesicles, where it forms NE. When an action potential in the neuron reaches the terminal, it causes NE to be released into the synapse. Following its action on receptors, the NE may be taken up by the neuron that released it, and it can then reenter the vesicle. NE not protected in the vesicle can be metabolized by monoamine oxidase (MAO). Both tricyclic antidepressants (TCAs) and MAO inhibitors (MAOIs) raise the synaptic concentration of NE.

The clinical effectiveness of these drugs is consistent with a hypothesis, developed in the late 1950s and early 1960s, theorizing that depression resulted from a deficiency in brain monoamines, either in their synthesis, release, metabolism, or removal, or in the sensitivity of the receptors for them (Schildkraut, 1965). This relatively straightforward hypothesis (monoamine hypothesis of depression, MAHOD) was also supported by clinical evidence that reserpine (Serpasil), an antihypertensive drug that depletes neurons of these same transmitters, can cause patients to become depressed or even suicidal. Thus, while reserpine is still available it is not a first-line drug to treat high blood pressure.

TRICYCLIC ANTIDEPRESSANTS (TCAs)

Another major class of drugs developed to treat depression is the tricyclic antidepressants (TCAs). Like the MAO inhibitors, these drugs were not initially developed to treat depression. In fact, they can be described as antihistamines "gone bad" (Domino, 1999). That is, they were developed as antihistamines, but they were not very good at stopping allergy symptoms and caused much too much drowsiness. However, TCAs definitely improved the mood of depressed patients. Interestingly, another failed attempt to develop a safe and effective antihistamine that did not cause drowsiness was chlorpromazine (Thorazine), an early and effective antipsychotic drug.

TCAs block the reuptake of NE and/or 5-HT into the neuron that released the neurotransmitter (Figure 2-3). Again, within the nervous system NTs are released by neurons into a synapse to act on other neurons or on smooth muscle, cardiac muscle, or exocrine glands. Blocking reuptake allows the NT to be in contact with its receptor at higher concentrations and for longer intervals than otherwise might occur. The effectiveness of these drugs on depression and their mechanism of action again were consistent with the somewhat vague monoamine hypothesis of depression (MAHOD) mentioned earlier.

The neuroanatomical locations of cells that produce NE and 5-HT as well as the locations of cells with NE and 5-HT receptors (with an assortment of subtypes) on them are consistent with the MAHOD.

SOURCES OF DEPRESSION

Understanding the roots of depression begins with looking at the neurotransmitter serotonin or 5-HT (Nestler, Hyman, & Malenka, 2008). Many cell bodies for neurons that synthesize 5-HT are located in the raphe nucleus in the midbrain (Figure 2-4). Where do the axons from the raphe nucleus project and what physiological functions and behaviors do these areas of the brain regulate? Axons from the raphe nucleus project to the frontal cortex, which regulates mood; to the basal ganglia, which helps control movements as well as obsessions and compulsions; to the limbic system, which appears to be involved in anxiety and panic; to the hypothalamus, which regulates (among many other functions) appetite and eating behavior; to the brainstem, which regulates sleep; and to the spinal cord, which controls several reflexes involved in normal sexual response (orgasm and ejaculation).

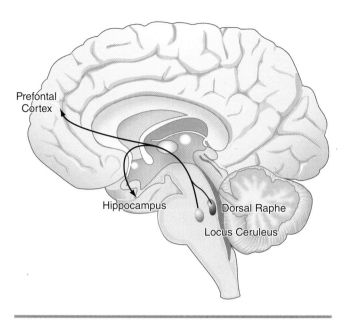

FIGURE 2-4 Serotonergic (5-HT) pathways from the dorsal raphe nucleus to the prefrontal cortex and the hippocampus and noradrenergic (NE) pathways from the locus ceruleus to the same regions are shown.

According to the MAHOD (Schildkraut, 1965), depression is due to a deficiency in some aspect of either NE or 5-HT activity in the brain. By looking at the neuroanatomy and neurophysiology just described, it is possible see how a 5-HT deficiency might result in symptoms of depression, anxiety, panic, phobias, obsessions, compulsions, and food cravings.

Norepinephrine (NE) pathways (Figure 2-4) also play a role in depression. Most cell bodies for NE-producing cells are located in an area of the brainstem known as the locus ceruleus. Projections from here go to the frontal cortex, where NE controls—or at least influences—mood, attention, concentration, working memory, and speed of information processing. Projections to the limbic system mediate emotions, feelings of energy, fatigue, psychomotor agitation, or psychomotor retardation. It is easy to see how a deficiency in brain NE activity might produce many of the characteristic symptoms of depression.

This analysis sounds logical but there is a huge hole in the hypothesis that can be articulated in one word: timing. All clinically useful antidepressants raise NE and/or 5-HT levels within a day or two (sometimes within hours), but clinical improvements may take 10 days to many weeks. If the symptoms of depression are due to a deficiency in NE or 5-HT activity in certain areas of the brain, and the antidepressants make their neurochemical repairs rather quickly, then why doesn't the depression go away just as quickly? This is in direct contrast to most other psychotropic medications. For example, after diazepam (Valium) interacts with its receptors in the brain, symptoms of anxiety usually diminish within an hour.

A somewhat newer theory is that the underlying neurochemical abnormality in depression is not with the NT per se, but with receptor activity or number. In this theory, reduced NT availability at the receptor leads to its up-regulation (i.e., an increase in the number of postsynaptic receptors for the NT). A study by Mann (Mann, Stanley, McBride, & McEwen,

1986) showed a 28% increase in the mean number of 5-HT2 receptors, and a 73% increase in beta-adrenergic receptor binding in the frontal cortex of patients who had committed violent suicide. However, while some studies have confirmed these findings (Yates et al., 1990), other studies have not.

Another real problem with both of these theories is that there is no clear-cut, consistent, reliable evidence of any measurable differences in the synthesis, release, uptake, metabolism, or receptor activity between depressed and euthymic patients for NE, 5-HT, or any other NT.

MULTISTEP PROCESSES

Newer theories go a step further, both figuratively and literally. Think of the relevant brain pathway involved in depression as a complicated device that it is designed to do what initially appears to be a simple task. Yet, this device, or brain pathway, is actually intricately equipped with multiple steps and levers. Imagine that everything at the start of the pathway (NT and its receptor) works perfectly but that a lever or step further along in the process is malfunctioning. In neurophysiology-speak, the problem is in signal transduction (Malberg & Blendy, 2005). That is, some step between the NT interacting with its receptor (the first step) and the maintenance of normal mood (a step much later in the process) is "broken" in depressed patients.

BRAIN-DERIVED NEUROTROPHIC FACTOR (BDNF) AND STRESS

A fairly new theory along these lines proposes that a triggering action, such as stress, interferes with the gene regulating brain-derived neurotrophic factor (BDNF), a vital neurochemical in the brain that helps maintain neuronal viability. Stephen Stahl (2008) described BDNF as fertilizer for brain cells. Neurotrophic factors, in general, are chemical substances in the brain that play a role in guiding nervous system development (Huang & Reichardt, 2001). While the developmental role has been recognized for some time, recent studies indicate that neurotrophic factors such as BDNF also play a critical role in the adult brain (Huang & Reichardt, 2001).

In theory, the lack of brain fertilizer, (i.e., reduced BDNF) allows certain vulnerable neurons in the hippocampus to atrophy and die, engendering the signs and symptoms of depression (Post, 2007; Schumacher et al., 2005) and, perhaps, Alzheimer's disease (Akatsu et al., 2006; Zhang et al., 2006). Several studies support this idea. In both rats and non-human primates, for example, chronic emotional and physical stress causes the death of hippocampal neurons (McEwen, 1999; Sapolsky, 1996). In human brain–imaging studies, hippocampal volume is measurably reduced in depressed patients (Duman, Malberg, & Thome, 1999). Moreover, expression of hippocampal BDNF is reduced in stressed animals (Smith, Makino, Kvetnansky, & Post, 1995).

Interestingly, both NE and 5-HT reuptake blockers used to treat chronic depression up-regulate expression (increase the amount produced) of both BDNF and its receptor in the rat hippocampus, and the timing of this up-regulation is consistent with the clinical improvement seen with these drugs (Xu et al., 2006). This effect appears to be specific to antidepressants in that non-antidepressant psychotropic drugs do not increase BDNF expression in this tissue. Several studies have reported similar findings in humans. In reports by Gorgulu & Caliyurt (2009) and Sen, Duman, & Sanacora (2008), serum BDNF levels were lower in depressed patients relative to healthy individuals and the levels normalized at times consistent with clinical improvement following drug therapy. Interestingly, Gorgulu & Caliyurt (2009) found that a single episode of total sleep deprivation for one full night elevated BDNF levels and significantly decreased symptoms of depression.

In summary, stress, a contributing factor for depression, causes a reduction in hippocampal volume, an effect observed in both animals and depressed humans. Stress also decreases hippocampal BDNF levels, and drugs used to treat depression increase BDNF levels at a time consistent with clinical improvement. These data all support the hypothesis that diminished BDNF may be a key contributing factor in depression and that raising its levels may be a common consequence of antidepressant therapy.

PHARMACOKINETICS

Antidepressant pharmacokinetics describes what the patient's body does with the drug, including how the drug is metabolized. Why is this so important in the treatment of depressed patients? Altered pharmacokinetics may help explain why some patients have "problems" with certain drugs (ineffectiveness or toxicity) and stop taking them (i.e., poor compliance).

For almost any depressed (unipolar or bipolar) patient, one of the first things the clinician will do is to conduct a thorough drug history that begins with noting what other drugs the patient is currently taking. It is likely that the depressed patient is already taking other drugs for a host of medical and nonmedical reasons. These may include drugs for diabetes, asthma, glaucoma, ulcers, insomnia, high blood pressure, and pain, as well as alcohol and tobacco. When two or more drugs are taken concurrently, they can interact with each other and produce undesirable side effects that may not occur when the drugs are taken individually. The more drugs the patient is taking, the higher the probability of a drug interaction (Brunton, Lazo, & Parker, 2006). One of the most important sources of drug interaction is competition for drug metabolizing enzymes, particularly the liver oxidative enzyme cytochrome P450 (CYP).

CYP is a key drug-metabolizing enzyme that is found primarily in the liver, although the intestinal form may also be relevant. CYP is actually an enzyme family with over 30 members, and each member has the ability to metabolize both naturally occurring chemicals (neurotransmitters, hormones, etc.) as well as drugs (Gonzalez & Tukey, 2006). Certain CYP members can metabolize lots of drugs, others a few, and some none at all. Having a sense of which drugs are metabolized by which CYP isozyme is useful in predicting and preventing harmful drug interactions that could interfere with treatment and outcomes.

Certain drugs such as the antidepressant fluvoxamine (Luvox) inhibit particular CYP isozymes (CYP1A2 and CYP3A4) whereas other drugs such as carbamazepine (Tegretol), an anticonvulsant and a mood stabilizer, can actually stimulate (induce) the formation of additional CYP. Depending on the other drug(s) the patient is taking, the blood level of the prescribed antidepressant may become too low to be clinically effective or so high as to produce symptoms of toxicity. There are many tables available that show which drugs are metabolized by which CYP isozyme and how likely it is to interact with antidepressant medications.

It is much more efficient to look up this information than to try and memorize it. First collect the patient's drug history, then, using a paper-, computer- or mobile-based drug guide, look for all major drug interactions with any drug that will be used. It is possible that two or more of the drugs that a patient is already taking are currently interacting to produce depression. Sometimes the best treatment is to subtract rather than add more drugs.

LIMITATIONS OF MAOIs AND TCAs

Until the development of the selective serotonin reuptake inhibitors (SSRIs), all earlier antidepressants (MAOIs and TCAs) had two critical limitations: there was a delay in onset of effect of at least 10 days to several weeks, and they are very toxic chemicals with therapeutic indices of between 5 and 15 (toxic to therapeutic dose) That is, as little as five times the therapeutic dose could be lethal. The incidence of suicide is significantly elevated in patients with mental illness. Approximately 10% to 15% of depressed patients are suicidal, and in schizophrenic patients suicide occurs at a rate as much as ten times higher than in the general population (Eisendrat & Lichtmache, 2009). The adverse effects of the MAOIs and TCAs can be described as the result of a "dumb" bomb. Although these drugs destroy their target (depression), they are nonselective and cause significant collateral damage; they have many severe and potentially lethal adverse effects (Table 2-1).

The biggest problem with the MAOIs is a potentially serious drug interaction with foods containing a naturally occurring chemical, tyramine. Although tyramine can cause peripheral neurons to rapidly release NE and the adrenal medulla to release epinephrine (adrenaline), dietary tyramine rarely has this effect because hepatic MAO normally breaks it down rapidly and efficiently.

What happens if a patient is taking a MAOI for depression? Under these conditions, the liver no longer metabolizes dietary tyramine and it is absorbed by the circulatory system. As it circulates, tyramine can increase NE release throughout the body (and epinephrine by the adrenal medulla) and can raise blood pressure (hypertension), increase heart rate (tachycardia), and cause seizures. Remember that MAO is the key intraneuronal enzyme that breaks down neuronal NE (Figure 2-3). When patients take a MAOI, it also raises neuronal NE levels, and if these patients eat foods rich in tyramine, both mechanisms can combine (i.e., intracellular NE levels are elevated by the MAOI and it is more easily released by the neuron due to the tyramine). The consequence is a massive release of NE, which can result in a hypertensive crisis, which could trigger a stroke. For this reason, foods containing tyramine

TABLE 2-1 Tricyclic Antidepressants: Sites of action vs. effects observed

TRICYCLIC ANTIDEPRESSANT ACTION	CLINICAL EFFECTS
Block reuptake of 5-HT and/or NE	Therapeutic effect
Block histamine (H1) receptor	Weight gain, drowsiness
Block muscarinic receptor	Dry mouth, blurred vision, constipation, drowsiness
Block alpha-1 receptor	Lightheadedness, decreased blood pressure
Block Na channels	Arrhythmias, cardiac arrest, and seizures

© Delmar/Cengage Learning

must be avoided by patients taking MAOIs. These foods include aged cheese, red wine, beer, broad beans (fava beans), bananas, avocados, yogurt, sour cream, and chocolate. There is also a potential lethal interaction when MAOIs are taken together with the opioid analgesic meperidine (Demerol) and several other drugs.

Patients taking TCAs frequently suffer a host of adverse effects. Some effects decline with time, and some are problematic throughout the duration of treatment. Most adverse effects result from the nonspecific action of TCAs at sites other than 5-HT or NE reuptake, which appears to be responsible for their antidepressant effects. For example, TCAs not only block reuptake of monoamines, they also block (1) muscarinic cholinergic receptors, (2) histamine-1 receptors, (3) alpha-1 adrenergic receptors at therapeutic concentrations, and (4) sodium channels in the heart and brain at toxic concentrations. A drug from this class must be taken for a minimum of three to four weeks just to see if it is effective, and it has a wide range of serious adverse effects and is potentially lethal in overdose. Moreover, because so many systems are affected by TCAs, overdoses (whether accidental or intentional) are particularly difficult to treat. As a result, health practitioners in emergency rooms settings dread treating people who have attempted suicide with TCAs (Ujhelyi, 1997).

SELECTIVE SEROTONIN REUPTAKE INHIBITORS (SSRIs)

Between the early 1960s and the late 1980s the state of affairs in antidepressants was "much ado about nothing." Then, in 1987, the FDA approved the use of fluoxetine (Prozac) for the treatment of depression (Vincent, 1994). Neurochemically, this drug almost exclusively blocks neuronal reuptake of 5-HT. Fluoxetine does not affect receptors for histamine, acetylcholine, serotonin, or norepinephrine, and it does not block sodium channels. It also does not significantly block the neuronal reuptake of norepinephrine. Fluoxetine was the first of a class of drugs known as selective serotonin reuptake inhibitors or SSRIs (Moore & Jefferson, 2004) and it was the first psychotropic smart bomb for depression. In marked contrast to earlier antidepressants, death due to overdose with drugs in this class is rare (in the absence of other drugs). As with the earlier drugs, clinical improvement is still delayed with SSRIs. The SSRIs also appeared to demonstrate the relative importance of manipulating 5-HT (rather than NE) levels in antidepressant action and strongly suggested that this monoamine was the key neurotransmitter underlying depression. Not only did fluoxetine open the door to an entirely new class of antidepressants, it indirectly led to the development of still other classes of antidepressants (Table 2-2).

TABLE 2-2 Example of Antidepressant Drugs, Categorized by Mechanism of Action

MAOIs	TCAs	SSRIs	DUAL-MECHANISM DRUGS
phenelzine (Nardil)	desipramine (Norpramin)	fluoxetine (Prozac)	venlafaxine (Effexor)
isocarboxazid (Marplan)	nortriptyline (Pamelor)	sertraline (Zoloft)	mirtazapine (Remeron)
tranylcypromine (Parnate)	amoxapine (Ascendin)	paroxetine (Paxil)	desvenlafaxine (Pristiq)
	maprotiline (Ludiomil)	fluvoxamine (Luvox)	buproprion (Wellbutrin)
	imipramine (Tofranil)	citalopram (Celexa)	
	clomipramine (Anafranil)	escitalopram (Lexapro)	
	amitriptyline (Elavil)		

© Delmar/Cengage Learning

While the SSRIs are clearly less toxic and better tolerated by patients, they are not without adverse effects, essentially all of which can be explained by the action of higher levels of 5-HT acting on one or more 5-HT-receptor subtypes in the brain, spinal cord, and GI tract (Azmitia & Whitaker-Azmitia, 1995). For example, stimulation of the 5-HT_{2A} and 5-HT_{2C} receptors (via elevated synaptic 5-HT levels) in the limbic system can cause mental agitation and anxiety or panic attacks. Action at 5-HT_{2A} receptors in the basal nuclei can affect motor movements whereas action at the same receptor subtype in the brainstem may disturb sleep and cause unwanted rapid muscle movements during the night. In the spinal cord 5-HT action on 5-HT_{2A} receptors can affect spinal reflexes necessary for orgasm and ejaculation, leading to sexual dysfunction. Action on 5-HT_3 receptors in certain areas of the brain can trigger nausea and vomiting and stimulation of 5-HT_3 or 5-HT_4 receptors in the gastrointestinal tract can produce cramps and diarrhea. Stahl (2008) refers to these (manageable) side effects as the "cost of doing business." Although SSRIs may be better tolerated than older drugs, they don't relieve depression any more rapidly than the older drugs. As with other antidepressants, clinical improvement following SSRI treatment may take weeks to be seen.

Norepinephrine Reuptake Inhibitors (NRIs)

Just as the essential role of 5-HT in depression and its treatment was starting to make some real sense, along came a new class of drugs, the selective norepinephrine reuptake inhibitors (NRIs), which, as the name implies, only inhibit the reuptake of NE. One drug in this class, reboxetine, is currently in use in Europe and seems to be at least as effective as the TCAs for treating depression (Papakostas, Nelson, Kasper, & Moller, 2008). So, which neurotransmitter is more important in depression and its effective treatment, 5-HT or NE?

Stahl (2008) points out that depression, in some patients, has characteristics of what might be seen with a "serotonin deficiency syndrome" (i.e., depression associated with anxiety, panics, phobias, posttraumatic stress disorder, obsessions, compulsions, or eating disorders), while others have characteristics of what might be seen with a "noradrenergic deficiency syndrome" (i.e., those whose depression is associated with fatigue, apathy, and notable cognitive disturbances, particularly impaired concentration, problems with sustaining and focusing attention, slowness in information processing, and deficiencies in working memory. This might explain why some patients do not respond to SSRIs or only partially respond (response but not remission). Only time will tell if certain patients will respond better to SSRIs while others respond better to NRIs.

In any case, the neural pathways associated with these two neurotransmitters have many opportunities to interact in several areas of the brain. In the frontal cortex, for example, where 5-HT neurons from the raphe nucleus synapse with other neurons, NE-containing neurons from the locus ceruleus also synapse close by. Interestingly, NE released by these neurons may interact with the 5-HT containing neurons and can inhibit the release of additional 5-HT (Figure 2-5).

At the somatodendritic end of the 5-HT neuron (near the cell body) in the raphe nucleus, NE can interact with alpha-1

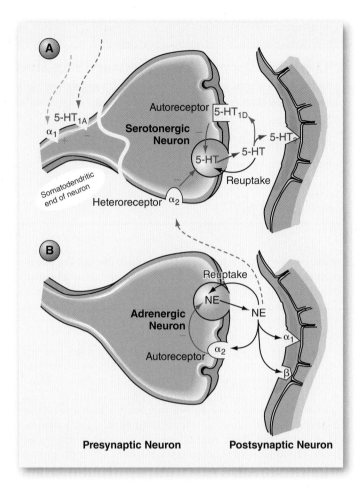

Figure 2-5 **Panel A: Serotonergic neuron. At the terminal end of the neuron (right) 5-HT is released and can act postsynaptically to trigger actions in an effector cell or it can act presynaptically on 5-HT_{1D} autoreceptors to inhibit additional 5-HT release. Also, NE from neighboring neurons can act on α_2 receptors to inhibit release of 5-HT. These are heteroreceptors. Finally a reuptake process can remove 5-HT from the synapse. At the dendritic end of the neuron (left), 5-HT can act on 5-HT_{1A} receptors inhibit the neuron while NE can act on α_2 receptors activating the cell.**

Panel B: Adrenergic neuron. At the terminal end of the neuron (right) NE is released and can act postsynaptically to trigger actions in an effector cell (α_1 or β receptors) or it can act presynaptically (α_2 receptors) or be taken back up by the neuron that released it.

receptors to increase activity along these neurons. In other words, norepinephrine can affect serotonin pathways and serotonin can affect norepinephrine pathways in the brain.

Selective Serotonin and Norepinephrine Reuptake Inhibitors (SNRIs)

Despite the safety of SSRIs, they are not always more effective than older antidepressants. In fact, remission rates with the TCAs are better than with SSRIs. This may be due to a

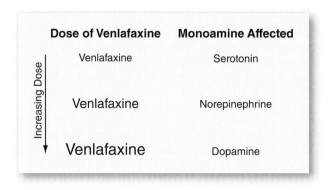

Dose of Venlafaxine	Monoamine Affected
Venlafaxine	Serotonin
Venlafaxine	Norepinephrine
Venlafaxine	Dopamine

(Increasing Dose ↓)

FIGURE 2-6 The antidepressant activity of venlafaxine may be mediated by three different monoamines, depending on dosage. At the lowest doses it only blocks the reuptake of 5-HT. At higher doses it also affects NE and the highest doses block the reuptake of dopamine (DA).

synergistic interaction between elevated 5-HT and NE. For treatment-resistant patients, two antidepressants are often taken simultaneously to gain from this synergy. Today, however, it is possible to get both actions from a single drug. Venlafaxine (Effexor) is one of several new dual- or multiple-mechanism antidepressants—that is, drugs that have antidepressant properties through two or more distinct mechanisms. Venlafaxine, at therapeutic doses, selectively blocks the reuptake of both serotonin and norepinephrine and at very high doses it also affects dopamine uptake (Figure 2-6) (Chen & Skolnick, 2007; Papakostas, Thase, Fava, Nelson, & Shelton, 2007). In 2008, the active metabolite of venlafaxine, desvenlafaxine (Pristiq) was approved by the FDA in a once-daily formulation for the treatment of adults with major depressive disorder. There is no evidence that it is any more effective than venlafaxine (Sopka, 2008), which coincidentally, goes off patent in 2010. These drugs may be abbreviated as SNRIs, selective serotonin and norepinephrine reuptake inhibitors.

If a single antidepressant raises both 5-HT and NE—and this is how the TCAs work (i.e., blocking 5-HT and NE reuptake)—then what is the advantage of the newer SNRIs over the older TCAs? Why don't drugs like venlafaxine have the same adverse effect profile as TCAs? Unlike the TCAs, venlafaxine does not affect adrenergic receptors, histaminergic receptors, or cholinergic receptors. It is the action of the TCAs on these receptors that trigger the vast majority of adverse effects caused by this class of drugs.

The most common adverse effect of venlafaxine, nausea, is greatly reduced when given in an extended-release (once daily) formulation. Other drugs acting via this same mechanism are currently under development. Venlafaxine, in addition to treating depression, is also an effective agent for generalized anxiety disorder, panic disorder, obsessive-compulsive disorder, social phobia, posttraumatic stress disorder, and bulimia (Gorman, 2003; Schoevers, Van, Koppelmans, Kool, & Dekker, 2008; Thase & Trivedi, 2002).

Whereas the efficacy of most antidepressants does not change as the dose is escalated (i.e., patients either improve or don't improve), raising the dose of venlafaxine improves efficacy (recovery > remission > response). Referred to by Stahl (2008) as a noradrenergic "boost," it occurs when the

second mechanism (blockade of NE reuptake) kicks in as the dose is raised. Stahl advocates the use of dual-mechanism antidepressants in patients who are resistant to SSRIs or in patients who respond to therapy but do not show remission of the illness.

Another dual-mechanism antidepressant is mirtazapine (Remeron). This drug is not a reuptake blocker for either NE or 5-HT. It is, however, a potent inhibitor of alpha-2 noradrenergic receptors (Clayton & Montejo, 2006). Alpha-2 receptors are located on both NE- and 5-HT-releasing neurons (Figure 2-5). This receptor provides negative feedback for the release of additional transmitter. To put it another way, when "enough" NE has been released by the neuron, some NE interacts with the presynaptic alpha-2 receptor, "alerting" the neuron to stop releasing NE. It is an autoreceptor or the neurochemical equivalent of a thermostat. In certain areas of the brain, such as the frontal cortex, where both serotonergic and noradrenergic terminals are in close proximity, alpha-2 receptors can be found on serotonergic neurons (Figure 2-5 part A), where they can reduce the release of 5-HT. Here, the alpha-2 receptor is referred to as a heteroreceptor (i.e., it regulates a neuron that releases a different neurotransmitter).

Since mirtazapine blocks this receptor on both adrenergic and serotonergic neurons, it turns off both inhibitory pathways. The effect of mirtazapine antagonism on presynaptic alpha-2 receptors is increased release of NE and 5-HT, resulting in SNRI-like clinical effectiveness. In addition to this primary action of mirtazapine, it also blocks 5-HT_{2A}, 5-HT_{2C}, and 5-HT_3 receptors, which, confusing as this may seem, turns out to be a good effect. These actions both enhance mirtazapine's antidepressant effectiveness and block some of the common adverse effects (such as anxiety, nausea, sexual dysfunction, and weight gain) of the SSRIs and SNRIs, which are the result of elevated 5-HT levels outside the central nervous system.

Bupropion (Wellbutrin) also has multiple actions on brain neurochemistry. It blocks both NE and DA uptake in the brain (Foley, DeSanty, & Kast, 2006; Wilkes, 2006). Bupropion has other uses as well, primarily for smoking cessation where is it sold under the brand name Zyban. It is effective for this condition because, in addition to its effects on NE and DA uptake, it is also an $\alpha_3\beta_4$ nicotinic receptor antagonist (Slemmer, Martin, & Damaj, 2000). Antagonism of this receptor appears to interrupt addiction, and it reduces the intensity of nicotine cravings and withdrawal symptoms following nicotine abstinence.

Another multiple mechanism drug is nefazodone (Serzone), which blocks 5-HT_{2A} receptors and is a selective serotonin and norepinephrine reuptake blocker (SNRI) (Pacher & Kecskemeti, 2004). So, while nefazodone increases both NE and 5-HT levels (in the brain and peripherally), it also blocks excessive 5-HT levels at the 5-HT_{2A} receptor. By doing so, nefazodone does not produce insomnia, anxiety, or sexual dysfunction usually associated with the SSRIs. In other words, the patient gets the benefits of an SSRI, with fewer adverse effects.

Despite this "apparent" advantage over other multiple mechanism antidepressants, once nefazodone began to be widely used for depression, reports of liver failure in treated patients started to appear. During all phases of clinical trials for a drug it is rare for more than 3,000 people to be exposed to a drug prior to its approval (or not) by the FDA. Thus, many adverse effects do not show up until the drug in widespread clinical use and many thousands of people have taken it. Even after a drug is approved, the FDA, in what is known as Phase IV or Post-Marketing Surveillance Trial, continues to check for rare adverse effects. Although the incidence of liver failure was rare (one case of liver failure resulting in death or transplant per 250,000–300,000 patient-years of nefazodone treatment, according to the manufacturer's Black Box warning), there was no way to predict which patients might develop this effect. In the end, the manufacturer voluntarily removed the drug from the European, Canadian and US markets in 2004.

DELAY IN SYMPTOM RELIEF

Most depressed patients are anxious for quick relief from their symptoms. Yet, despite the advances in antidepressant drug therapy in the past half-century, all clinically available antidepressants, regardless of mechanism, have a delay in onset of relief from weeks to months. However, a study with an older drug gives promise to the idea that rapid onset antidepressants may yet be developed. Large scale clinical trials with ketamine are currently under way. Zarate and coworkers (Zarate et al., 2006) reported that a single dose of ketamine, an intravenous anesthetic and a "club drug," significantly improved symptoms of depression in treatment-resistant depressed patients (DSM-IV major depression) in less than two hours. The improvement, moreover, was significant throughout the next seven days. Could ketamine be the Holy Grail of antidepressant therapy because just one dose results in rapid onset and long-lasting effect? Before jumping to any conclusions, be sure to read the Zarate article.

So how does Special K (ketamine's street name) fit in? Ketamine is an NMDA-receptor antagonist. The NMDA receptor is a subtype of receptor for glutamate, an excitatory neurotransmitter in the brain. The Zarate study and other data (Paul & Skolnick, 2003) suggest that altered glutamate function may be closer to the underlying neurobiological disturbance that causes depression, whereas the monoamines may be several steps back or to the side in the process and that the delayed therapeutic success for drugs acting via monoamines is due to the eventual disruption of this glutamate pathway.

In summary, if the drugs acting via monoamines might be considered as steps A or B in the model of depression, then perhaps the NMDA receptor is step K or L, closer to the final goal of symptom relief.

Other downstream steps in this process—and, thus, targets for rational antidepressant drug development—include a veritable alphabet soup of naturally occurring brain chemicals. These include CRH (corticotropin releasing hormone), Ca^{2+} (calcium), NO (nitric oxide), CREB (cyclic AMP response element binding protein), and BDNF (brain-derived neurotrophic factor). The final step appears to be increased neurogenesis in the hippocampus and certain other brain regions (such as the frontal cortex), resulting in the relief of depression.

The onset of action of essentially all antidepressant drugs is delayed for up to several weeks, since they require adaptive changes downstream of the initial neuromolecular event,

while numerous factors interplaying and interacting with each other may (or may not) contribute toward depression and its treatment. According to this hypothetical model (Figure 2-7), depression occurs if certain factors, such as intense ongoing stress, mediated by CRH, leads to a decrease in cellular production of BDNF, a critical neurotrophic factor in the brain (Anisman, 2009; Marini, Popolo, Pan, Blondeau, & Lipsky, 2008; Yulug, Ozan, Gonul, & Kilic, 2009). Neurotrophic factors are protein growth factors within the brain that assure the survival of neurons. When hippocampal BDNF is diminished, as has been reported in both humans and in animal models of depression, apoptosis (programmed cell death) increases, and neuroplasticity and neurogenesis of certain neuron populations in this region decline. With chronic depression, the hippocampus actually shrinks in volume (Schmidt & Duman, 2007; Smith et al., 1995).

Chronic—but not acute—treatment with 5-HT and/or NE uptake blockers (SSRIs, SNRIs, TCAs), however, has been shown to increase intracellular BDNF gene expression and BDNF levels (Vaidya & Duman, 2001). This is accompanied by an antiapoptotic effect (i.e., cells do not die off as easily), as well as increased neuroplasticity and increased neurogenesis in the hippocampus. In some ways, this goes against traditional thinking, which holds that brain cell production (i.e., neurogenesis) does not take place after birth. Following this line of reasoning, once hippocampal brain cells die during depression, all treatment should capable of is preventing further loss, not growing replacement neurons. But the sprouting of hippocampal cells (granule cells and mossy fibers) does occur in adults following antidepressant drug treatment (Schmidt & Duman, 2007).

√BDNF'S ROLE

Brain-derived neurotrophic factor, or BDNF, appears to play a crucial and essential role in normal and abnormal brain function, in mental health, and in mental illness. Figure 2-7 shows how several neurotransmitters interact with their receptors and a common outcome is the elevation of BDNF synthesis and release. Its role in the onset and treatment of depression is clearest and perhaps best characterized. BDNF is also discussed in later chapters that cover bipolar disorder, psychosis, and Alzheimer's disease.

Release of BDNF from granules in central nervous system neurons, particularly in the hippocampus and frontal cortex (Lipska, Khaing, Weickert, & Weinberger, 2001) can be enhanced or diminished by numerous factors. Two key pathways involved in its release are mediated by the intracellular second messengers cAMP and CAM kinase (Figure 2-7; abbreviations are in figure legend). Each of these pathways can be activated by both NE and 5-HT, although via different receptor subtypes. Even though the model in Figure 2-7 implies that all the receptors illustrated are on or in the same cell, this is generally not the case.

For example, on certain cell membranes the β-adrenergic receptor for NE or the 5-$HT_{4,6,7}$-receptor subtypes for serotonin elevate cellular cAMP levels, which subsequently activates the enzyme PKA. Likewise, on other neurons, NE acting at the α_1 receptor or 5-HT acting on the 5-HT_2 receptor elevates the intracellular messenger protein CAM-kinase, which increases CREB. In both cases, either through increased PKA

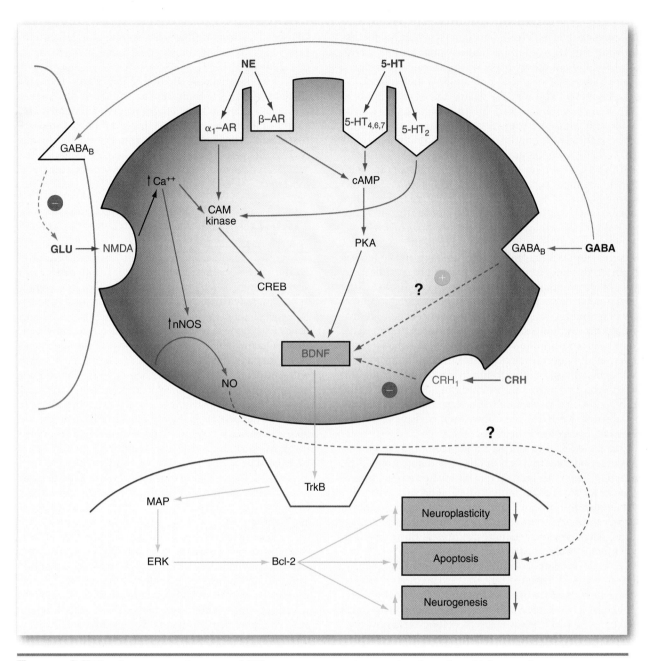

FIGURE 2-7 This demonstrates how several different neurotransmitters, acting through multiple second-messenger systems, can increase the levels of BDNF, which appears to be neuroprotective.

Abbreviations:

α_1–AR — Alpha-1-adrenoceptor
β–AR — Beta-adrenoceptor
Bcl-2 — Beta cell lymphoma 2
BDNF — Brain derived neurotrophic factor
CREB — cAMP response element binding protein
cAMP — Cyclic adenosine monophosphate
CAM — Ca^{2+}/calmodulin dependent protein kinase
CRH — Corticotropin releasing hormone
ERK — Extracellular signal regulated protein kinase

GABA — Gamma amino butyric acid
GLU — Glutamate
MAP — Mitogen-activated protein (kinase)
NMDA — N-methyl-D-aspartate
NO — Nitric oxide
nNOS — Neural nitric oxide synthase
PKA — cAMP dependent protein kinase
TrkB — Tyrosine kinase B

or increased CREB activity, the neurons begin to produce and release more BDNF. It is important to remember that essentially all antidepressant medications raise either or both NE and 5-HT levels but with a delay in clinical improvement of about 10 days to two weeks, minimum. Which transmitter is more important and why the delay? The slow increase in the synthesis and release of BDNF may explain why raising brain levels of either transmitter can improve the symptoms of depression—assuming, of course, that BDNF activity is actually related to depression.

BDNF is one of several neurotrophic factors in brain that each act at a unique receptor. BDNF acts at the TrkB receptor (Figure 2-7) (Tsai, 2006). Stimulating this receptor produces numerous cellular events via a potpourri of 3- and 4-letter abbreviations for ineffable intracellular messengers. TrkB receptor activation produces three highly significant effects: neuroplasticity (neuroadaptability), neurogenesis (growth of new neurons), and apoptosis (programmed cell death). Neuroplasticity reflects the brain's ability to adapt to a wide range of changing conditions, insults, and injuries and is essential for learning and memory to occur. Neurogenesis is the generation or regeneration of brain tissue, once thought to occur in its entirety before birth. To a certain degree, however, neurogenesis continues throughout life, especially in areas of the brain involved in learning and memory (the hippocampus, for example). Activation of the TrkB receptor also slows apoptosis, programmed cell death. It now known that BDNF can slow—and perhaps reverse—this process in certain brain cells.

Chronic stress, a key contributing factor in many major depressive disorders that acts via the stress hormone CRH, lowers BDNF levels (Figure 2-7). Diminished stimulation of the TrkB receptor results in decreased neuroplasticity (difficulty learning and remembering), as well as in increased apoptosis and decreased neurogenesis (loss of hippocampal volume). Antidepressant therapy can reverse these effects in animal models of chronic stress.

An important neurotransmitter involved in learning and memory is glutamate (GLU). It is the most common excitatory neurotransmitter in the brain. But raising GLU levels can be a two-edged sword. When its concentration is somewhat elevated, it allows a key step, long-term potentiation (LTP), to occur along the molecular pathway for learning (Shapiro, 2001). When that happens, repeated, intense synaptic firing across the same pathway (which occurs during learning) leads to chemical and structural changes in neurons that facilitate future activity along that pathway (the event is remembered). This appears to take place through calcium (perhaps via CAM kinase to sequentially elevate CREB and BDNF, Figure 2-7). However, if BDNF and intracellular calcium levels are too high, then it can be neurotoxic (Calabresi, Centonze, & Bernardi, 2000). This is likely due to increased synthesis of nitric oxide (NO), a very small neurotransmitter molecule that diffuses from one cell to the next. Too much NO can have neuronal effects exactly opposite of what is described above for BDNF (Dawson, 1995). That is, NO can decrease neuroplasticity, decrease neurogenesis, and increase apoptosis or cell death.

The potential role of GLU in depression is fascinating, since ketamine, the injectable anesthetic mentioned earlier, is a selective and potent GLU-receptor antagonist (NMDA subtype). However, it also is a powerful hallucinogen. Given that stimulating the NMDA receptor (with GLU) increases NO levels, which increases apoptosis, it is logical that an NMDA antagonist such as ketamine should quickly reverse this effect.

DEPRESSION: PAST AND PRESENT ⚡

In the past 50 years, the thinking about depression has changed from viewing it as a character flaw to recognizing it as an illness with an underlying neurochemical disturbance. Moreover, clinicians have gone from having only a handful of drugs with poor margins of safety and serious adverse effects to now having a wide array of drugs that are safer to use and easier for patients to tolerate. Today, more patients are treated with antidepressants than ever before. In fact, antidepressants are among the most widely prescribed drugs in the United States. Unfortunately, there are still no clinically effective drugs for depression that work quickly. All currently available medications can take up to several weeks to work and they don't all work in all patients. Ongoing research appears to be elucidating the key neurochemical steps and neuroanatomical loci of depression. As these potential targets for intervention are better understood, more effective drugs with fewer adverse effects and more rapid onset of action will be forthcoming.

Three recent articles show that, despite all of our advances in the past half-century, there are still many controversial issues to resolve when it comes to depression and antidepressant therapy. For example, once recent meta-analysis of clinical data by Mykletun and coworkers (2009) suggest that the danger of depression may be higher than earlier thought. The authors report that depression-associated mortality is comparable to that of cigarette smoking. While such an analysis might suggest more aggressive and earlier treatment of depression, another study by Turner and coworkers (2008) suggests that data from clinical trials on a variety of antidepressant drugs with negative outcomes tend not to get published whereas those with positive outcomes are almost always published. Since this is partly how the FDA decides whether or not to approve a drug, the inherent bias of such a system makes it difficult to determine a drug's true clinical efficacy. Lastly, a study by Fournier et al., published this year (2010) suggests that antidepressants are no better than placebo for mild, moderate, or severely depressed patients, but are clearly effective in patients with very severe symptoms.

REVIEW QUESTIONS

1. In order to claim that a depressed patient is in remission, what conditions must be met?
   a. Patient is symptom free for 7 to 10 days
   b. Patient has no more than two episodes of (unipolar or bipolar) depression for six months following initiation of treatment with an SSRI
   c. Patient remains symptom free for up to one year
   d. Patient must be symptom free for one to three months following termination of drug treatment

2. What is the biggest flaw associated with the monoamine hypothesis of depression (MAHOD), which states that depression is due to a deficiency in the production, storage, or release of monoamine neurotransmitters or there is altered/diminished sensitivity to them by their associated receptors?
   a. It does not account for the action of the SSRIs.
   b. The MAHOD can only explain how an antidepressant affects a single neurotransmitter, whereas newer drugs, such as venlafaxine (Effexor) can affect multiple neurotransmitters.
   c. If the MAHOD was correct, clinical improvement should occur within hours, not weeks.
   d. The MAHOD assumes only a single receptor subtype for each neurotransmitter.

3. When bupropion is used to treat depression, it sold under the brand name Wellbutrin. What else may it be used to treat and under what brand name is it sold?
   a. Hair regrowth; Rogaine
   b. Erectile dysfunction; Viagra
   c. Smoking cessation; Zyban
   d. Schizophrenia; Abilify

4. Which of the following drugs has been shown, in small clinical trials, to reduce the symptoms of depression within an hour?
   a. Ketamine (Ketalar)
   b. Mirtazapine (Remeron)
   c. Lithium carbonate (Lithobid)
   d. Escitalopram (Lexapro)

5. What neurotrophic factor in the hippocampus is reduced in depressed patients and can be elevated with antidepressant treatment?
   a. Adrenocorticotrophic hormone (ACTH)
   b. Brain derived neurotrophic factor (BDNF)
   c. Corticotrophic releasing (factor) hormone (CRH)
   d. Benzodiazepine neurotrophic releasing factor (BNRF)

6. Match the following behavior effects with sites in the CNS at which 5-HT is elevated due to the action of SSRIs such as fluoxetine.

Frontal cortex	a. orgasm and ejaculation
Basal ganglia	b. appetite and eating behavior
Hypothalamus	c. movement
Spinal cord	d. mood

7. Why is BDNF referred to as brain "fertilizer"?
   a. It is high in nitrogen content.
   b. It increases neurogenesis, enhances neuroplasticity, and slows down apoptosis.
   c. Before it changed to BDNF, this neurotrophic factor went by the acronym FTLZR, which is pronounced fertilizer.
   d. An adverse effect of drugs acting through this neurotrophic factor is severe diarrhea.

8. What was the major clinical advantage gained with the advent of SSRIs such as fluoxetine (Prozac) in the late 1980s?
   a. Longer action, less frequent dosing, and better compliance
   b. Significantly higher remission rates than with TCAs or MAOIs
   c. Because of its limited sites of action, they do not affect receptors for NE, 5-HT, ACh, and Histamine, and death due to overdose is rare.
   d. In contrast to older antidepressants, the opioid antagonist naloxone (Narcan) can be used to reverse an overdose of an SSRI.

9. What is a potential clinical advantage of using venlafaxine (Effexor XR), a drug that blocks the reuptake of BOTH 5-HT and NE, over the use of SSRIs or TCAs?
   a. Unlike the older drugs, venlafaxine is without adverse effects.
   b. In treatment resistant depressed patients, using a single drug that acts through more than one mechanism may be beneficial due to synergy.
   c. The combined effect of the elevated 5-HT and NE leads to an increase in DA (dopamine) levels and rapid mood elevation.
   d. Whereas TCAs and SSRIs often take three to four weeks to attain clinical effectiveness, mood improvement is seen within three days with venlafaxine.

10. What does the injectable anesthetic ketamine do that no other drug has been shown to do before?
    a. Be equally effective in both phases of bipolar mood disorder
    b. Allows the patient to remain in a dissociative state until depression recedes
    c. The same dose given intravenously can also be given orally to treat depression, implying that there is absolutely no metabolism or excretion until after it has reached and acted upon the NMDA receptor in brain.
    d. In small controlled clinical studies it has been shown to improve symptoms of depression in treatment-resistant depressed patients in less than two hours.

REFERENCES

Akatsu, H., Yamagata, H. D., Kawamata, J., Kamino, K., Takeda, M., Yamamoto, T., et al. (2006). Variations in the BDNF gene in autopsy-confirmed Alzheimer's disease and dementia with Lewy bodies in Japan. *Dementia & Geriatric Cognitive Disorders, 22*(3), 216–222.

Anisman, H. (2009). Cascading effects of stressors and inflammatory immune system activation: Implications for major depressive disorder. *Journal of Psychiatry & Neuroscience, 34*(1), 4–20.

Azmitia, E. C., & Whitaker-Azmitia, P. M. (1995). Anatomy, cell biology, and plasticity of the seronergic system. In F. E. Bloom & D. L. Kupfer (Eds.), *Psychopharmacology: The fourth generation of progress* (pp. 443–449). New York: Raven Press.

Brunton, L. L., Lazo, J. S., & Parker, K. L. (2006). Principles of Toxicology and treatment of poisoning. In L. S. Goodman, A. Gilman, L. L. Brunton, J. S. Lazo, & K. L. Parker (Eds.), *Goodman & Gilman's the pharmacological basis of therapeutics* (11th ed.). New York: McGraw-Hill.

Calabresi, P., Centonze, D., & Bernardi, G. (2000). Cellular factors controlling neuronal vulnerability in the brain: A lesson from the striatum. *Neurology, 55*(9), 1249–1255.

Chen, Z., & Skolnick, P. (2007). Triple uptake inhibitors: Therapeutic potential in depression and beyond. *Expert Opinion on Investigational Drugs, 16*(9), 1365–1377.

Clayton, A. H., & Montejo, A. L. (2006). Major depressive disorder, antidepressants, and sexual dysfunction. *Journal of Clinical Psychiatry, 67*(Suppl 6), 33–37.

Dawson, V. L. (1995). Nitric oxide: Role in neurotoxicity. *Clinical & Experimental Pharmacology & Physiology, 22*(4), 305–308.

Domino, E. F. (1999). History of modern psychopharmacology: A personal view with an emphasis on antidepressants. *Psychosomatic Medicine, 61*(5), 591–598.

Duman, R. S., Malberg, J., & Thome, J. (1999). Neural plasticity to stress and antidepressant treatment. *Biological Psychiatry, 46*(9), 1181–1191.

Eisendrat, S. J., & Lichtmache, J. E. (2009). Psychiatric disorders. In S. J. McPhee, M. A. Papadakis, & L. M. Tierney Jr. (Eds.), *Current medical diagnosis & treatment* (48th ed.). New York: McGraw-Hill.

Foley, K. F., DeSanty, K. P., & Kast, R. E. (2006). Bupropion: Pharmacology and therapeutic applications. *Expert Review of Neurotherapeutics, 6*(9), 1249–1265.

Fournier, J. C., DeRubeis, R. J., Hollon, S. D., Dimidjian, S., Amsterdam, J. D., Shelton, R. C., & Fawcett, J. (2010). Antidepressant Drug Effects and Depression Severity: A Patient-Level Meta-analysis. *JAMA, 303*(1), 47–53.

Gonzalez, F. J., & Tukey, R. H. (2006). Drug metabolism. In L. S. Goodman, A. Gilman, L. L. Brunton, J. S. Lazo, & K. L. Parker (Eds.), *Goodman & Gilman's the pharmacological basis of therapeutics* (11th ed.). New York: McGraw-Hill.

Gorgulu, Y., & Caliyurt, O. (2009). Rapid antidepressant effects of sleep deprivation therapy correlates with serum BDNF changes in major depression. *Brain Research Bulletin, 80*(3), 158.

Gorman, J. M. (2003). Treating generalized anxiety disorder. *Journal of Clinical Psychiatry, 64*(Suppl 2), 24–29.

Healy, D. (1997). *The antidepressant era.* Cambridge, Mass.: Harvard University Press.

Huang, E. J., & Reichardt, L. F. (2001). Neurotrophins: Roles in neuronal development and function. *Annual Review of Neuroscience, 24*, 677–736.

Kroenke, K. (2003). Patients presenting with somatic complaints: Epidemiology, psychiatric co-morbidity and management. *International Journal of Methods in Psychiatric Research, 12*(1), 34–43.

Lipska, B. K., Khaing, Z. Z., Weickert, C. S., & Weinberger, D. R. (2001). BDNF mRNA expression in rat hippocampus and prefrontal cortex: Effects of neonatal ventral hippocampal damage and antipsychotic drugs. *European Journal of Neuroscience, 14*(1), 135–144.

Malberg, J. E., & Blendy, J. A. (2005). Antidepressant action: To the nucleus and beyond. *Trends in Pharmacological Sciences, 26*(12), 631–638.

Mann, J. J., Stanley, M., McBride, P. A., & McEwen, B. S. (1986). Increased serotonin2 and beta-adrenergic receptor binding in the frontal cortices of suicide victims. *Archives of General Psychiatry, 43*(10), 954–959.

Marini, A. M., Popolo, M., Pan, H., Blondeau, N., & Lipsky, R. H. (2008). Brain adaptation to stressful stimuli: A new perspective on potential therapeutic approaches based on BDNF and NMDA receptors. *CNS & Neurological Disorders Drug Targets, 7*(4), 382–390.

McEwen, B. S. (1999). Stress and hippocampal plasticity. *Annual Review of Neuroscience, 22*, 105–122.

Moore, D. P., & Jefferson, J. W. (2004). Selective serotonin reuptake inhibitors. *Moore & Jefferson: Handbook of medical psychiatry* (2nd ed.). Philadelphia, Pa: Mosby Elsevier.

Mykletun, A., Bjerkeset, O., Øverland, S., Prince, M., Dewey, M., & Stewart, M. (2009). Levels of anxiety and depression as predictors of mortality: The HUNT study. *The British Journal of Psychiatry, 195*, 118–125.

Nestler, E. J., Hyman, S. E., & Malenka, R. C. (2008). *Molecular neuropharmacology: A foundation for clinical neuroscience* (2nd ed.). New York: McGraw-Hill.

Papakostas, G. I., Nelson, J. C., Kasper, S., & Moller, H. J. (2008). A meta-analysis of clinical trials comparing reboxetine, a norepinephrine reuptake inhibitor, with selective serotonin reuptake inhibitors for the treatment of major depressive disorder. *European Neuropsychopharmacology, 18*(2), 122–127.

Papakostas, G. I., Thase, M. E., Fava, M., Nelson, J. C., & Shelton, R. C. (2007). Are antidepressant drugs that combine serotonergic and noradrenergic mechanisms of action more effective than the selective serotonin reuptake inhibitors in treating major depressive disorder? A meta-analysis of studies of newer agents. *Biological Psychiatry, 62*(11), 1217–1227.

Paul, I. A., & Skolnick, P. (2003). Glutamate and depression: Clinical and preclinical studies. *Annals of the New York Academy of Sciences, 1003,* 250–272.

Post, R. M. (2007). Role of BDNF in bipolar and unipolar disorder: Clinical and theoretical implications. *Journal of Psychiatric Research, 41*(12), 979–990.

Rakel, R. E., & Bope, E. T. (2008). Mood disorders. *Conn's current therapy* (60th ed.). Philadelphia: Saunders Elsevier.

Sapolsky, R. (1996). Stress, glucocorticoids, and damage to the nervous system: The current state of confusion. *Stress, 1,* 1–19.

Schildkraut, J. J. (1965). The catecholamine hypothesis of affective disorders: A review of supporting evidence. *American Journal of Psychiatry, 122*(5), 509–522.

Schmidt, H. D., & Duman, R. S. (2007). The role of neurotrophic factors in adult hippocampal neurogenesis, antidepressant treatments and animal models of depressive-like behavior. *Behavioural Pharmacology, 18*(5–6), 391–418.

Schoevers, R. A., Van, H. L., Koppelmans, V., Kool, S., & Dekker, J. J. (2008). Managing the patient with co-morbid depression and an anxiety disorder. *Drugs, 68*(12), 1621–1634.

Schumacher, J., Jamra, R. A., Becker, T., Ohlraun, S., Klopp, N., Binder, E. B., et al. (2005). Evidence for a relationship between genetic variants at the brain-derived neurotrophic factor (BDNF) locus and major depression. *Biological Psychiatry, 58*(4), 307–314.

Selikoff, I. J., & Robitzek, E. H. (1952). Tuberculosis chemotherapy with hydrazine derivatives of isonicotinic acid. *Diseases of the Chest, 21*(4), 385–438.

Sen, S., Duman, R., & Sanacora, G. (2008). Serum brain-derived neurotrophic factor, depression, and antidepressant medications: Meta-analyses and implications. *Biological Psychiatry, 64*(6), 527–532.

Shapiro, M. (2001). Plasticity, hippocampal place cells, and cognitive maps. *Archives of Neurology, 58*(6), 874–881.

Slemmer, J. E., Martin, B. R., & Damaj, M. I. (2000). Bupropion is a nicotinic antagonist. *Journal of Pharmacology & Experimental Therapeutics, 295*(1), 321–327.

Smith, M. A., Makino, S., Kvetnansky, R., & Post, R. M. (1995). Stress and glucocorticoids affect the expression of brain-derived neurotrophic factor and neurotrophin-3 mRNAs in the hippocampus. *Journal of Neuroscience, 15*(3 Pt 1), 1768–1777.

Stahl, S. M. (2008). *Stahl's essential psychopharmacology: Neuroscientific basis and practical applications* (3rd ed.). New York: Cambridge University Press.

Thase, M. E., & Trivedi, M. (2002). Optimizing treatment outcomes for patients with depression and generalized anxiety disorder. *Psychopharmacology Bulletin, 36*(Suppl 2), 93–102.

Tsai, S. J. (2006). TrkB partial agonists: Potential treatment strategy for epilepsy, mania, and autism. *Medical Hypotheses, 66*(1), 173–175.

Turner, E. H., Matthews, A. M., Linardatos, E., Tell, R. A., & Rosenthal, R. (2008). Selective publication of antidepressant trials and its influence on apparent efficacy. *N Engl J Med, 358,* 252–260.

Ujhelyi, M. R. (1997). Assessment of tricyclic antidepressant toxicity: Looking for a needle in a pharmacologic haystack.[comment]. *Critical Care Medicine, 25*(10), 1634–1636.

Vaidya, V. A., & Duman, R. S. (2001). Depression—emerging insights from neurobiology. *British Medical Bulletin, 57,* 61–79.

Vincent, J. D. (1994). [Biology of pleasure]. [La biologie du plaisir.] *Presse Medicale, 23*(40), 1871–1876.

Wilkes, S. (2006). Bupropion. *Drugs of Today, 42*(10), 671–681.

Xu, H., Chen, Z., He, J., Haimanot, S., Li, X., Dyck, L., et al. (2006). Synergetic effects of quetiapine and venlafaxine in preventing the chronic restraint stress-induced decrease in cell proliferation and BDNF expression in rat hippocampus. *Hippocampus, 16*(6), 551–559.

Yates, M., Leake, A., Candy, J. M., Fairbairn, A. F., McKeith, I. G., & Ferrier, I. N. (1990). 5HT2 receptor changes in major depression. *Biological Psychiatry, 27*(5), 489–496.

Yulug, B., Ozan, E., Gonul, A. S., & Kilic, E. (2009). Brain-derived neurotrophic factor, stress and depression: A minireview. *Brain Research Bulletin, 78*(6), 267–269.

Zarate, C. A., Jr., Singh, J. B., Carlson, P. J., Brutsche, N. E., Ameli, R., Luckenbaugh, D. A., et al. (2006). A randomized trial of an N-methyl-D-aspartate antagonist in treatment-resistant major depression. *Archives of General Psychiatry, 63*(8), 856–864.

Zhang, H., Ozbay, F., Lappalainen, J., Kranzler, H. R., van Dyck, C. H., Charney, D. S., et al. (2006). Brain derived neurotrophic factor (BDNF) gene variants and Alzheimer's disease, affective disorders, posttraumatic stress disorder, schizophrenia, and substance dependence. *American Journal of Medical Genetics.Part B, Neuropsychiatric Genetics: The Official Publication of the International Society of Psychiatric Genetics, 141*(4), 387–393.

CHAPTER 3
Pharmacotherapy of Bipolar Disorder

"It is sayd there be a raunge of mountaynes in the Easte, on one syde of the which certayn conducts are immorall, yet on the other syde they are holden in good esteeme; wherebye the mountayneer is much conveenyenced, for it is given to him to goe downe eyther way and act as it shall suite his moode, withouten offence." Gooke's Meditations

AMBROSE BIERCE

GETTING PERSONAL

When I was in my early 20s I moved into my own apartment. It was an exciting move for me, however, during the first year of living on my own, my emotions took a tumultuous ride and I learned that I was bipolar.

My mania came first, and it lasted for more than six months. During that time, I was full of energy every day, even though I was getting very little sleep at night. I frequently had racing thoughts, where my mind seemed to be working in overdrive to take in and process information. Because of my racing thoughts, I felt I had all the answers. I began to develop overly ambitious and grandiose ideas and some days, I would obsess over them for hours. I was experiencing a new level of confidence and anything I wanted seemed easily and quickly attainable. At the same time however, I was becoming very irritable and edgy. When a close friend or family member would disagree with me, I would become very defensive and sometimes would go off the deep end.

Then it all came crashing down. There was such a quick and dramatic change in my mood, from manic to depressive, that I can remember the week it happened. During that week, I began questioning every aspect of my confidence and my whole world was turned upside down. For the next four or five months, I was consumed by depression and almost every week, I seemed to hit a new low. Along with my depression came anxiety, which also seemed to only get worse. As it went on, all I had were negative thoughts and I lost any hope of things getting better.

I did seek help from several doctors and was diagnosed with bipolar disorder, but unfortunately the doctors were unable to help me. The day finally came when I called my dad and told him I was ready to end it all. After talking about ending things for months, he knew I really meant it this time, and he urged me to check into a hospital. At that point, I was ready to take the step and go into inpatient treatment.

Going into the hospital was nothing like what I expected and it was certainly one of the best decisions I've ever made. From that day forward, everything has been better. In the hospital, I had a team of psychiatrists talking with me every day. After discussing my symptoms at length, they put me on a combination of mood stabilizing medicines. When I left the hospital, I found a highly recommended psychiatrist and during my first few sessions we talked about my state of mind and made several adjustments to the dosages of my medicine to better stabilize my mood, which keeps me from feeling the highs of mania and the lows of depression.

Without the support of my parents and the doctors who have helped me, my life's story might have ended tragically. I owe everything to them.

Anonymous

BIPOLAR MOOD DISORDER

The term *bipolar mood disorder* is relatively new. For example, in the mid-1850s in France, the term used to describe the disease was *olie à double forme* (dual-form insanity) or the equally politically incorrect term *folie circulaire* (circular insanity). The respected German psychiatrist Emil Kraepelin (1856–1926), the father of modern psychiatry, coined the term "manic-depressive insanity" in the late 1800s (Healy, Harris, Farquhar, Tschinkel, & Le Noury, 2008). However, the very name of this illness automatically conferred a stigma on the patient who was unlucky enough to be symptomatic. In the 1960s, another German scientist, Karl Leonhard, recognized that the key distinguishing feature of the illness was its polarity and classified affective disorders as being unipolar or bipolar (Perris, 1990). This description made it quite simple to switch the name of the disorder to the more neutral term, bipolar mood disorder. In 2000, according to the World Health Organization, bipolar disorder was the ninth leading cause of disability in the world (WHO, 2001), affecting between 1.1% and 6% of the general population (Kessler et al., 2006).

Depression can be unipolar or bipolar (Figure 3-1). In unipolar depression, patients experience one or more episodes of depression during their lifetime. With a bipolar mood disorder, however, some patients experience bouts of mania interspersed among the episodes of dysthymia. While manic, patients often have feelings of amplified energy,

extremely elevated mood (euphoria), rapid speech, racing thoughts, decreased need for sleep, hypersexuality, grandiosity, and excessive interest in goal-directed activities. The symptoms of mania range from mild impairment in judgment and insight (hypomania) to such a level of excitement and dysfunction that hospitalization is required in order to regain control. Delusions and hallucinations, characteristic symptoms of psychosis, may accompany these manic episodes. Because of these additional symptoms, bipolar mood disorders are much more difficult to treat than unipolar depression and multiple-drug therapy is standard, rather than optional.

When patients are manic they have very high energy levels, and they have thoughts racing through their minds. They make decisions in a flash and spend less and less time sleeping. They may describe themselves as feeling "high as a kite," and seem to be excessively optimistic in anything they try. These patients can become highly irritable and are often impatient with others. They frequently engage in inappropriate, impulsive, and risky behaviors. Their ideas, to them at least, are exceedingly creative, with their senses highly attuned to their surroundings. For the patient who is manic, everything seems to be connected in ways only they can appreciate. During acute manic episodes, patients may experience delusions (fixed, false, irrational, or illogical beliefs) and hallucinations (hearing, seeing, or sensing things without there being a stimulus to cause them).

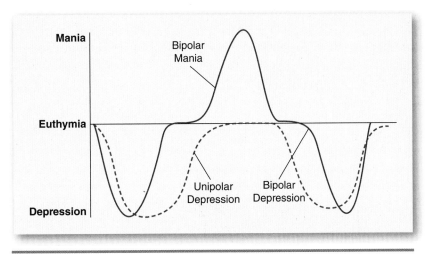

FIGURE 3-1 Unipolar Depression and Bipolar Disorder. Time course of unipolar (dashed line) depression and bipolar mood disorder (solid line).

BIPOLAR CATEGORIES

Based on the criteria specified in DSM-IV TR (American Psychiatric Association, 2000), patients with bipolar disorders fall into one of four diagnostic categories (Figure 3-2): bipolar I, bipolar II, cyclothymia, and "bipolar disorder not-otherwise specified," depending on the symptoms. A key element in the bipolar classification is the current or past history of at least one manic episode. Also, in contrast to the traditional psychiatric notion that a bipolar patient, at the time of presentation, is *either* manic *or* depressed (or euthymic), it is now recognized that some patients may simultaneously display some symptoms of depression and some symptoms of mania. This blended presentation of symptoms is a mixed episode. The following information provides a brief review each of these categories, since diagnosis may help with the treatment decision. To delve more deeply into these diagnostic criteria, refer to the DSM-IV guidelines or a textbook that is more focused on diagnostic aspects of mood disorders.

Patients with Bipolar I disorder are distinct from other bipolar patients in that their clinical course has been marked by the appearance of one or more manic episodes or mixed episodes. Whereas some patients present with their first and only (reported) manic episode, others have had a history of mood disorders. In this regard, DSM-IV describes six distinct subtypes of Bipolar I disorders, generally based on the most recent (current) episode: (1) Single Manic Episode, (2) Most Recent Episode Hypomanic, (3) Most Recent Episode Manic, (4) Most Recent Episode Mixed, (5) Most Recent Episode Depressed, and (6) Most Recent Episode Unspecified. Moreover, many of these patients have also had one or more Major Depressive Episodes during their lives. Since the symptoms of Bipolar I Disorder may be secondary rather than primary, one must first exclude diagnoses such as a Substance-Induced Mood Disorder (due to the direct effects of a medication, other somatic treatments for depression, a drug of abuse, or toxin exposure) or Mood Disorder Due to a General Medical Condition.

The patient's presenting symptoms and history of mood disorders are shown graphically in Figure 3-2 (Panels A–F) for each of these six subclasses of Bipolar I Disorder. Also shown are the mood profiles of patients with Bipolar II Disorder (Panel G) and with Cyclothymic Disorder (Panel H).

BIPOLAR I SUBTYPES
Single Manic Episode (Figure 3-2, A)

These patients have no previous history of diagnosed mood disorders and are experiencing their first manic episode. DSM-IV TR describes a manic episode as "a distinct period during which there is an abnormally and persistently elevated, expansive, or irritable mood . . . [that] must last at least 1 week."

Most Recent Episode Hypomanic (Figure 3-2, B)

Hypomania's characteristic symptoms are identical to those of mania but are not severe enough to markedly impair social or occupational functioning or require hospitalization, and thus do not meet the diagnostic criteria for mania. Patients with this subtype of Bipolar I Disorder present as hypomanic and have had a prior history of at least one manic episode or mixed episode. Moreover, at the time of diagnosis, the patient's mood symptoms are severe enough that they have begun to affect social and occupational functioning.

Most Recent Episode Manic (Figure 3-2, C)

These patients present with a manic episode and have had a prior history of one or more manic, major depressive or mixed episodes.

Most Recent Episode Mixed (Figure 3-2, D)

These patients present with a mixed episode and have had a prior history of one or more manic, major depressive or mixed episodes.

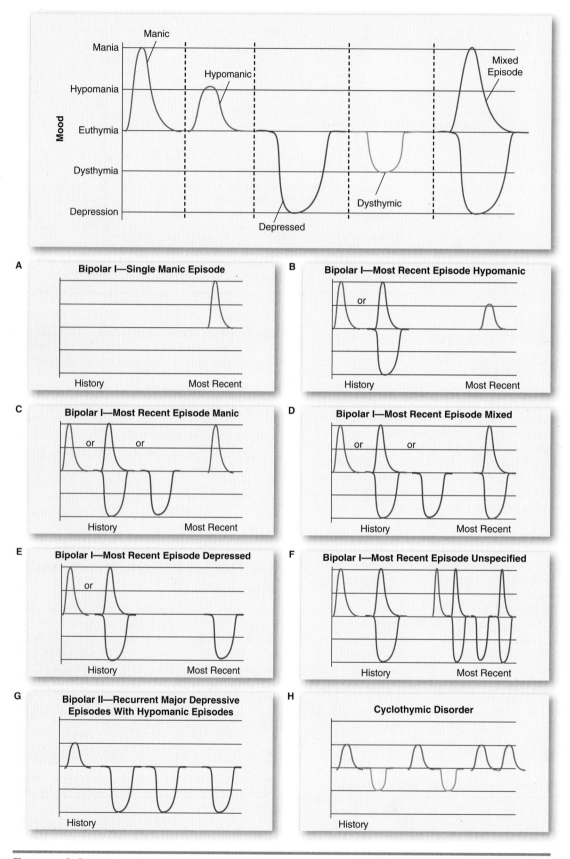

FIGURE 3-2 Bipolar Mood Disorders. The top panel shows the ways in which bipolar disorder may be manifest as mania, hypomania, depression, dysthymia and as a mixed episode. Panels A–F describe six distinct subtypes of Bipolar I disorders, generally based on the most recent (current) episode: (A) Single Manic Episode, (B) Most Recent Episode Hypomanic, (C) Most Recent Episode Manic, (D) Most Recent Episode Mixed, (E) Most Recent Episode Depressed, and (F) Most Recent Episode Unspecified. Also shown are the mood profiles of patients with Bipolar II Disorder (Panel G) and with Cyclothymic Disorder (Panel H).

Most Recent Episode Depressed (Figure 3-2, E)

These patients present with a major depressive episode and have had a prior history of one or more manic, or mixed episodes. The history of a prior major depressive episode is not an option, since there must be some evidence of mania, either at present or in the past to meet the criteria of Bipolar Disorder.

Most Recent Episode Unspecified (Figure 3-2, F)

These patients present with symptoms of a manic episode, a major depressive episode, or a mixed episode but do not meet the duration criteria for any of them. These patients also have a prior history of a manic episode or a mixed episode.

BIPOLAR II (FIGURE 3-2, G)

Patients with Bipolar II disorder have had one or more major depressive episodes and at least one hypomanic (not manic) episode. Patients who have had one or more manic or mixed episodes in the past, but are presenting with a major depressive episode or a hypomanic episode would be categorized as having Bipolar I—Most Recent Episode Depressed (Figure 3-2, E), or Bipolar I—Most Recent Episode Hypomanic (Figure 3-2, B), rather than Bipolar II.

✓CYCLOTHYMIA (FIGURE 3-2, H)

Cyclothymic disorder is characterized by repeated episodes of hypomanic and dysthymic symptoms over a two-year period in which there have been no diagnosed episodes of major depression. In addition, the number, severity, pervasiveness, or duration of symptoms is insufficient to meet the criteria for mania or major depression. Put simply, cyclothymic disorder is milder form of bipolar disorder.

One thing should be clear from the above descriptions of Bipolar Disorder subtypes; it is not possible to accurately diagnose a patient based solely on the presenting symptoms. A patient, who, for example, presents with symptoms of major depression, may have a Major Depressive Disorder or may have a Bipolar I or Bipolar II disorder. This distinction can only come from obtaining an accurate patient history.

Not all patients fit so neatly into one of these two classes. Some patients have to deal with (or endure) rapid cycling, experiencing mood swings several times per day or at least four or more mood swings in a 12-month interval, while other patients have mixed episodes in which certain symptoms of both mania and depression coincide. Sometimes a patient's bipolar symptoms make it difficult to choose one of the specific diagnosable categories of DSM-IV (American Psychiatric Association, 2000). For these patients, a new catchall category has cropped up, Bipolar-NOS (Not Otherwise Specified).

The problem with the Bipolar-NOS category is that rather than being a miscellaneous classification for the few cases that do not fit the traditional classes of bipolar disorder (Bipolar I or II), it actually includes the majority of all cases of bipolar mood disorders. Kessler (2006) noted that the prevalence of Bipolar I Disorder in the adult population is about 0.8% and the prevalence of Bipolar II Disorder is about 1.1%, whereas current clinical and epidemiologic evidence suggest that actual prevalence of all bipolar spectrum disorders, including Bipolar Disorder-NOS, is approximately 6%.

Since the late 1990s, H. S. Akiskal has published over 300 articles, mostly on bipolar disorder. In a systematic manner Akiskal suggests additional categories including:

- Bipolar II½—Cyclothymic depressions
- Bipolar III—Antidepressant-associated hypomania
- Bipolar III½—Bipolarity masked—and unmasked—by stimulant abuse
- Bipolar IV—Hyperthymic depression

Stahl (2008) expands this spectrum still further describing the appearance of patients with bipolar ¼ and bipolar ½, bipolar I½, bipolar II½, bipolar V, and bipolar VI. The major advantage of such a system is that it allows for consistent and precise descriptions of observed behaviors; it allows clinicians to diagnose a patient as bipolar without being restricted to just two categories or having to utilize the clumsy term Bipolar Disorder-NOS, which implies "my clinical experience tells me the patient is bipolar even though he or she doesn't fit the DSM-IV TR (2000) guidelines."

Although the incidence of bipolar disorder may be lower than other psychiatric disorders, these patients, compared to other psychiatric patients, are more likely to attempt suicide. When it comes to pharmacotherapy, bipolar patients present special challenges. Not only must clinicians treat the depression, they also must treat the manic episodes when they appear, and must consider the use of prophylactic therapy during euthymic periods to prevent mood swings from occurring in either direction. Even with intensive treatment, approximately two-thirds of bipolar patients remain moderately to severely ill throughout the year (Suppes, Kelly, & Perla, 2005).

Perhaps the fastest-growing population diagnosed with bipolar mood disorder includes children and adolescents. From 1995 to 2000 the number of patients under the age of 20 who received outpatient treatment for bipolar disorder rose 67% while the number who received inpatient treatment rose by 74% (Moreno et al., 2007). This is likely due to the increased diagnosis and treatment of this illness in children and adolescents. Yet, there is also a disturbing third option—that the disorder is being overdiagnosed and overtreated in this population. At this point the answer is not clear.

DEPRESSION THERAPIES

When treating a patient with bipolar mood disorder there are three important issues to consider: What type of therapy is used to treat episodes of depression; what is used to treat mania; and what is used to stabilize patients' moods while they are euthymic. In general, three classes of drugs are utilized in this patient population. These include (1) lithium carbonate, (2) anticonvulsants, and (3) atypical antipsychotics. One particular class of drugs that is normally used to treat unipolar depression, antidepressants, is not included on this list.

Based on the discussion on depression, it might seem like treating an episode of depression in bipolar patients with an antidepressant is the logical choice and for many years it was—and too often, still is. However, when given alone (i.e., monotherapy) antidepressants are likely to be a poor choice for treating bipolar patients. There is a large body of evidence showing that, in the absence of a mood stabilizer, antidepressants can rapidly switch a patient's mood from depression to mania (treatment-emergent mania) and accelerate mood cycling (Wehr & Goodwin, 1979). The bulk of this evidence, however, was collected with tricyclic antidepressants (TCAs) and monoamine oxidase inhibitors (MAOIs). Recent studies with SSRIs suggest that they are less likely than older drugs to induce a mood switch, especially if coadministered with a mood stabilizer (Grunze, 2005).

A PHARMACEUTICAL INVENTORY

In general, the question is not whether to treat patients with bipolar disorder but when to treat them, and with which drug(s). In the course of the illness, there are two windows for prescribing mood stabilizers. One window occurs when treating the bipolar patient for the first time, often during an acute manic episode when the disorder is often first diagnosed. The other opportunity occurs when they are euthymic. This prophylactic treatment—while the patient is asymptomatic—makes bipolar disorder somewhat different from other psychiatric illnesses.

LITHIUM

The word *lithium* is derived from the Greek word *lithos* meaning "stone." Lithium, the other white salt, is a simple element that has many characteristics of sodium. In fact, in the mid-1940s lithium chloride became a popular salt substitute for patients on sodium-free diets. Its importance in psychiatry was immediately recognized following a study by Cade (1949). Cade found lithium to be effective in all 10 of the manic patients he treated, but it was ineffective in patients with dementia praecox (schizophrenia) or chronic depressive psychosis. Since then hundreds of studies have confirmed his findings and extended them, showing that chronic treatment with lithium carbonate (Eskalith, Lithobid) not only helps abbreviate a manic episode; it also actually prevents mood swings in either direction, up or down. Recently a study by Ohgami et al. (2009) demonstrated that even minuscule levels of lithium that show up in municipal drinking water could lower that community's risk of suicide. In other words, lithium is the prototypic mood stabilizer.

While it is clear that lithium works, there is no good answer as to how or why it works. Earlier, when lithium was only used for manic episodes, proponents of the MAHOD (monoamine hypothesis of depression) believed that lithium had the opposite effect of antidepressants on NE and/or 5-HT synthesis, release, metabolism, and reuptake or receptor sensitivity. That is, lithium decreased activity in one of these "excessively" functioning pathways. But once lithium was shown to be effective in preventing both mania and depression, it no longer neatly fit into the MAHOD. If anything, lithium (by deceasing monoamine activity) should have worsened depression, not improved it.

Current theories of lithium action focus on postsynaptic cellular signaling mechanisms, after the neurotransmitter interacts with its receptor. Lithium is an inhibitor of a key enzyme essential in intracellular signaling (Watson & Young, 2001). Recent data suggest that, among other actions, lithium alters this signaling pathway by beginning a process that ends

with increased hippocampal neurogenesis, neuroplasticity, and cell survival in the hippocampus (Foland et al., 2008; Fukumoto, Morinobu, Okamoto, Kagaya, & Yamawaki, 2001; Shaltiel, Chen, & Manji, 2007). This is consistent with the theory discussed in the last chapter, that depression may be triggered by a deficiency in BDNF leading to atrophy or cell death of certain vulnerable neurons in the hippocampus (as well as other areas in the brain).

Although about 80% of manic patients respond to acute lithium treatment, it is a challenging drug to work with as it has a narrow therapeutic dose range (0.6–1.2 mEq/L). Lithium is limited by its adverse effects, which often appear at therapeutic concentrations (0.8–1.4 mEq/L) (Freeman & Freeman, 2006). These effects include fatigue, muscular weakness, slurred speech, ataxia, fine tremor of the hands, and excessive thirst and urination. At toxic concentrations (>2 mEq/L), consciousness is impaired and coma may result. Lithium toxicity is dramatically increased in the presence of a low-salt diet, as the kidneys make a valiant but counterproductive effort to retain sodium. Frequently, hypertensive patients or those concerned about weight gain and bloating go on low-salt diets or take medications that increase sodium excretion. This can cause serious complications of the patient is also taking lithium. The clinician must be aware of these circumstances before prescribing this drug (McNamara, 2006).

ANTICONVULSANTS

Anticonvulsants are normally used to treat and prevent seizures in patients with epilepsy. For the past 20 years, however, two anticonvulsants, carbamazepine (Tegretol) and valproic acid (Depakote) have also been used with bipolar patients as alternatives to lithium for mood stabilization. Another, newer anticonvulsant, lamotrigine (Lamictal), is also effective and was approved by the FDA for maintenance treatment of bipolar disorder in 2003 (Grunze, 2005).

It is not known how anticonvulsants work to prevent mood swings. The one thing these three drugs have in common is that they inhibit the sodium channels that are activated when the cell is receiving neuronal signals (i.e., use-dependent or voltage-gated channels) (McNamara, 2006). The more activity the cell is receiving, the more these channels are activated, which is a key step in triggering an action potential. By inactivating voltage-gated sodium channels, the anticonvulsants prevent the spread of high-frequency abnormal electrical signals to areas in the brain other than at the source. In other words, they protect the brain against seizures. Altering these channels also inhibits the excitatory brain transmitter glutamate (GLU) and activates the inhibitory transmitter gamma-aminobutyric acid (GABA).

Not all anticonvulsants are effective as mood stabilizers. For example, the older anticonvulsants phenytoin (Dilantin) and phenobarbital are ineffective. Newer anticonvulsants have also been evaluated with mixed results. Gabapentin (Neurontin) and topiramate (Topamax) have limited utility because of toxicity, the need for frequent administration, and the delayed onset of efficacy. Three of the most recent FDA-approved anticonvulsants—levetiracetam (Keppra), zonisamide (Zonegran), and tiagabine (Gabitril)—have not yet been fully evaluated (i.e., double-blind clinical trials) as mood stabilizers (Goldberg & Citrome, 2005).

While adverse effects are much less likely to appear with this class of drugs than with lithium, they are not without side effects (McNamara, 2006). Valproic acid, for example, may cause hair loss, weight gain, and sedation. In women of childbearing age it may increase the risk of birth defects and menstrual disturbances, and it can cause obesity and insulin resistance. Carbamazepine may cause sedation and hematological abnormalities. Common adverse effects of lamotrigine include dizziness, sleepiness, headache, visual disturbances, nausea, vomiting, and rash. One type of rash (Stevens-Johnson syndrome) caused by lamotrigine, although rare (incidence of 0.8%), may be life threatening and requires hospitalization.

ANTIPSYCHOTICS

Classic antipsychotic drugs, such as haloperidol (Haldol) and chlorpromazine (Thorazine) have been used for decades to help manage patients during episodes of agitation and psychosis in acute mania. In the last few years, newer, atypical antipsychotics such as olanzapine (Zyprexa) and quetiapine (Seroquel) have been used effectively in treating and preventing depression in bipolar patients (Calabrese et al., 2005).

What is an atypical antipsychotic and what makes it atypical? Until a little more than a decade ago, all antipsychotic drugs had a common adverse effect. They frequently caused debilitating motor problems with symptoms identical to those seen in Parkinsonism. New antipsychotic drugs developed over the last 20 years, while structurally diverse, are far less likely to produce these (extrapyramidal) motor side effects than are the older drugs. They are, in other words, atypical antipsychotics.

Antipsychotic drugs (covered in greater detail in Chapter 4) are clinically effective because they block possibly abnormal dopamine (DA) receptors in select areas of the brain. The atypical antipsychotics also block these receptors and they block certain 5-HT receptor subtypes particularly 5-HT_{2A} that the older drugs did not affect. How exactly blocking 5-HT receptors prevents a clearly identified DA-mediated side effect is less clear. Mood stabilization achieved by blocking 5-HT_{2A} receptors might reasonably be expected to improve depression. After all, this is precisely the mechanism of action of mirtazapine (Remeron) a newer antidepressant. It is possible, as well, that the DA antagonist action of these drugs not only gives them antimanic properties, but may also play a role in stabilizing mood (Dunlop & Nemeroff, 2007). Some of the adverse effects that atypical antipsychotics may produce include drowsiness, dry mouth, dizziness, and constipation.

Atypical antipsychotic drugs that have been FDA-approved for treatment of bipolar mania include clozapine (Clozaril), olanzapine (Zyprexa), risperidone (Risperdal), quetiapine (Seroquel), ziprasidone (Geodon), and aripiprazole (Abilify) (Gajwani et al., 2006). These drugs may be used as monotherapy or as adjuncts to lithium or valproate treatment. In 2004 olanzapine was the first atypical antipsychotic to be approved to treat bipolar mania and mixed episodes, and it was the first atypical antipsychotic drug approved for bipolar maintenance treatment. A combination drug containing both olanzapine and fluoxetine (Symbyax) is also approved for treatment of bipolar depression (Deeks & Keating, 2008).

ELECTROCONVULSIVE THERAPY (ECT)

A highly effective nonpharmacologic treatment for bipolar depression is electroconvulsive therapy (ECT). Because ECT has a rapid onset of action, it provides a viable alternative to drug treatment for patients with severe or psychotic depression, particularly in patients who are at high risk for suicide or in patients who are intolerant to drugs. But it is not clear just how ECT works. There is some evidence that BDNF may be involved, since chronic ECT up-regulates expression of BDNF and its receptor TrkB. Both ECT and lithium increase neurogenesis in the hippocampus and select other areas of the brain (Duman, Nakagawa, & Malberg, 2001). In fact, the reduced gray-matter volume in human prefrontal cortex that is seen in untreated bipolar patients is not observed in lithium-treated subjects (Moore, Bebchuk, Wilds, Chen, & Manji, 2000).

POTENTIAL ROLE OF BDNF

BDNF seems to have a role in all forms of mental illnesses and their cures. As in depression, BDNF appears to play a crucial role in both the etiology of bipolar disorder and in the effects of the mood stabilizers, particularly lithium. However, the precise role of BDNF in bipolar disorder is not clear. There is evidence that the amount of BDNF present is less important than is its trafficking in the neuron (post-translational processing) and release in response to nervous system activity.

MOLECULAR BIOLOGY BASICS

Chapter 2 discusses BDNF and its potential role in depression and, in particular, with hippocampal function and dysfunction. BDNF also seems to be involved in both bipolar disorder and in schizophrenia, although in far more subtle ways. The following information provides a brief molecular biology primer to give some background and perspective on how genetic information is translated into the structure and function of the body.

All proteins (e.g., BDNF) are produced by a process that begins at the level of the gene (Figure 3-3), a meticulous and consistent sequence of nucleic acids on a chromosome. Humans have 23 pairs of chromosomes, containing over 50,000 genes, about half of which code for proteins. A chromosome consists of two intertwined strands of nucleic acids. A nucleic acid in one strand is paired with and weakly bound to a specific nucleic acid in its helically twisted opposing strand. The human genome contains over 3 billion base pairs (Human Genome Program, 1992). An adenine molecule on one strand is paired with thymine in the opposite strand, and a cytosine molecule pairs with guanine. Each sequence of three nucleic acids (a codon) represents one of 20 possible amino acids. Amino acids link to each other to form a protein.

When an "appropriate" stimulus arrives at the nucleus and a gene is activated, one strand of DNA unzips or unwinds from the other and is used as a template to create messenger-RNA (mRNA). The mRNA emerges from the nucleus and moves to the ribosome where it is paired up with transfer-RNA (tRNA).

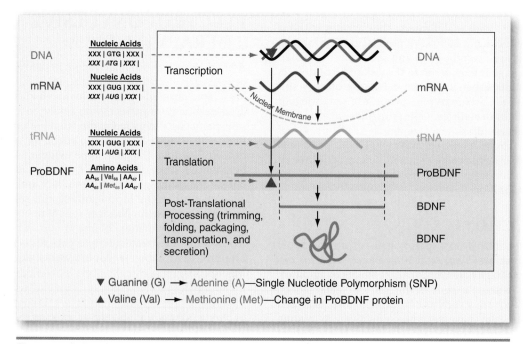

FIGURE 3-3 BDNF Gene Transcription. Due to a genetic mutation in a single locus, in which a guanine nucleotide is replaced by adenine, the resulting protein ends up with a methionine instead of valine at codon 66 in the BDNF precursor protein, proBDNF. This molecule is cleaved to form a "normal" BDNF molecule, which is then released by the neuron.

The ribosome uses the tRNA as a blueprint to fabricate the desired protein, which is then cleaved to the correct length, neatly folded into a bundle, packaged into a cellular envelope, and then transported to other parts of the cell. In the case of a neuron, the molecule may be carried to the nerve terminal where it can be released. Based on a predesignated signal, the protein is released into the synapse to do its job. This process varies to a degree across all living cells, and some proteins are used within the cell to maintain its normal health, structural integrity, or function.

With so many steps and so many molecules it is easy for things to go awry, and it often does. Genetic mutations in living organisms are extremely common and although some are fatal to a cell or to the organism itself, many mutations produce end products no different from the intended protein or at least ones that are not harmful to the organism. Most, in fact, provide organisms with the variety of life. When more than one variant of a specific gene is found in a population, it is referred to as *polymorphism*. Common human polymorphisms include gender (male, female), blood type (A, B, AB, and O), and eye color (brown, blue, green). There are literally hundreds of thousands of single base pair variations—single nucleotide polymorphisms or SNPs—in the 3 billion base pair human genome. Many medical conditions, including mental illnesses, may have a genetic basis or at least may occur in people with a genetic predisposition. It is hoped that identifying gene variants in "diseased" versus healthy subjects will help to identify the genetic basis of many disease states, which should lead to more effective treatments.

Two other important terms are *homozygous* and *heterozygous*. Humans have 23 pairs of chromosomes, with half of

each pair contributed by one parent and half by the other. If the gene contributed by each parent is the same, the person is said to be homozygous for that gene. If the gene contributed by each parent does not match exactly, the gene is said to be heterozygous.

So just where does BDNF fit in when it comes to genetics? Interestingly, it is in the middle ring of this molecular biology three-ring-circus. One of the most common BDNF polymorphisms (SNP) occurs at a very specific locus on the gene (nucleotide 196) where instead of the guanine (G) nucleotide appearing, adenine (A) insinuates itself (see Figure 3-3). As this "typo" is transcribed into RNA and then translated into the protein BDNF, the error is perpetuated . . . sort of, and this is where the story gets interesting. In the protein proBDNF, the error is such that valine (Val), the amino acid that should be made, is replaced by methionine (Met). This occurs at the 66th amino acid in the proBDNF protein sequence. There are two chances of getting the gene right or wrong, since one gene comes from the mother and the other from the father. Possible variants of the gene include Val66Val (both standard), Val66Met (one standard and one with the SNP), and Met66Met (both with SNP), depending on whether both parents supplied a Val or Met variant or one parent supplied one variant while the other parent supplied the alternate.

Often, when a protein is expressed or translated, it is longer than it needs to be and the end (or ends) must be snipped off. Think of a candle that is manufactured with an extra-long wick. Before the candle leaves the factory, any extra wick is removed. For BDNF, the protein produced by the ribosome is proBDNF (Seidah, Benjannet, Pareek, Chretien, & Murphy, 1996), and this protein needs to be trimmed before it can be released. Val66Met (or Met66Met), when it occurs, is in the part of the proBDNF molecule that is cleaved off and the final BDNF produced is identical to the predominant form of the protein (Val66Val). It looks and acts the same as "normal" BDNF, because it is exactly the same; only the cleaved-off portion is different and that is very, very important.

BDNF VARIANTS

BDNF in adults is a critical component of normal neural processes involved in synaptic plasticity, dendritic growth, and long-term memory consolidation. In the hippocampus, an area of the brain vital to learning and memory, BDNF is secreted in response to increased neuronal activity. Its release from postsynaptic dendrites is activity dependent and may be a key component of hippocampal-based synaptic plasticity and long-term potentiation (LTP), a key step in learning and memory (Egan et al., 2003).

So, does a single amino acid mutation in the cleaved-off portion of proBDNF play a role in learning and memory and bipolar mood disorders? As noted earlier, the biological activity of BDNF released by both gene variants is identical. What is not identical is the amount released in response to electrical activity in the hippocampus, and this difference in release may contribute to differences in learning and memory and the appearance of certain psychiatric disorders (Fan & Sklar, 2008; Post, 2007).

Compared to healthy human test subjects with the Val66Val form of the gene (i.e., the phenotype in which both parents contribute the predominant variant of the gene), those with Val66Met polymorphism displayed significant decreases in memory performance (Hariri et al., 2003), as well as decreased hippocampal volume and increased activation during learning and memory assessment (Bueller et al., 2006; Egan et al., 2003). Egan also reports that people with the Val66Met or Met66Met variant had specific difficulties with episodic or working memory (e.g., Where were you and what were you doing on the night of January 23, 2004?). And those people with Met66Met had the greatest difficulty with working memory (Egan et al., 2003).

Obviously parents, if they had the option, would want their children to have the Val66Val variant, so that they are "normal" and equipped with the best genes possible for learning and memory. The assumption is that with these genes their children will get into the best schools and will be a valedictorian—but then again, maybe not.

Several studies have looked at the association between particular BDNF variants and mental illness, including bipolar disorder. Of the 12 studies that examined the relationship with bipolar, 7 found a positive association between the presence of the Val66Val allele and the incidence of this disorder (Geller et al., 2004; Green et al., 2006; Lohoff et al., 2005; Neves-Pereira et al., 2002; Skibinska et al., 2004; Sklar et al., 2002), while 5 studies found no association (Hong, Yu, Lin, & Tsai, 2003; Kunugi et al., 2004; Nakata et al., 2003; Neves-Pereira et al., 2005). It is possible that the differences in findings among these studies may be due to sampling differences, in that the positive association studies were all done on North American or British patients and the negative association studies were done in Asian or other populations. The highest

association between the Val66Val BDNF and bipolar disorder occurred in two subsets: those with early onset (Skibinska et al., 2004) and those with the rapid cycling form of the disorder (Green et al., 2006).

This begs the question as to whether BDNF plays a role in bipolar disorder or not. The answer is a simple straightforward . . . maybe. Whereas people with the Val66Val allele may have memory problems, increased hippocampal activity, decreased gray matter in some cortical areas, and perhaps a higher incidence of schizophrenia, it is not associated with bipolar disorder (and in fact may be protective for bipolar onset). On the other hand, an association has been found in persons with the Met allele—either Val66Met or Met66Met—particularly in the incidence of early onset (18 years or younger) bipolar disorder (Skibinska et al., 2004).

But if the BDNF produced by the Val and Met variants is the same, then what accounts for the differences in these two phenotypes? It appears that the Met variant of the ProBDNF molecule, from which BDNF is derived, is not released or is not cleaved as easily as the Val variant following an increase in neuronal activity, such as might occur when the brain is trying to learn something new. Thus, the same amount of brain stimulation would result in less BDNF being released in the Met variants, which might explain cognitive dysfunction. Why the Val66Val allele is associated with bipolar disorder is not readily understood.

TAILORING TREATMENT

Just as a child is not a small adult when it comes to drug therapy, the bipolar patient is not merely a depressed patient with extra symptoms. It both cases, drug treatment must be tailored to meet the patient's special needs. Treating bipolar patients with a TCA, a MAOI, or an SSRI when they are depressed may cause them to swing quickly into a manic state (polarity switch), so these drugs should not be used alone in bipolar patients (Ali & Milev, 2003). Along with any antidepressant drugs patients are taking, a mood stabilizer should also be taken to minimize the possibility of a polarity shift.

Many drugs are available to treat acute mania. These include lithium and most antipsychotics, particularly if the patient is highly agitated or psychotic. The anticonvulsants valproic acid and carbamazepine may also be used.

Perhaps the single most important aspect in the pharmacological management of the bipolar patient is stabilizing the patient's mood during euthymic periods, when the patient is not manic, hypomanic, or depressed. Successful management means fewer hospitalizations and suicides and better patient quality-of-life reports.

For many years, the only mood stabilizer available to bipolar patients was lithium, the standard to which other drugs are still compared. Lithium use is limited by toxicity, which often occurs at therapeutic doses. Some patients cannot or will not tolerate this drug. Approximately 66% of patients on lithium are noncompliant.

Over time, certain anticonvulsants (valproic acid and carbamazepine) began to be used as alternatives to lithium when it was ineffective or could not be tolerated. For a while, lamotrigine (Lamictal) was the most widely investigated anti-convulsant for the treatment of bipolar disorder. In the 2002 revised American Psychiatric Association practice guidelines, lamotrigine was recommended as a first-line treatment of acute mania in bipolar depression, and in 2004 the FDA approved it for maintenance treatment of bipolar disorder. Interestingly, it now appears that lamotrigine is more effective in preventing depressive symptoms than in treating mania (Calabrese et al., 2008). Not all anticonvulsants are equally effective. Older drugs just do not seem to work and newer ones have not been adequately studied (Gajwani et al., 2005).

Another class of drugs that has found its way into the treatment of bipolar patients is the atypical antipsychotics. Several such drugs, which were first used in bipolar patients for acute manic episodes, are now used as mood stabilizers.

Treating the bipolar patient can be a clinician's nightmare. While the manic symptoms scream for attention, the depressive symptoms are more insidious, as most bipolar patients spend at least 50% of their lives under the shadow of depression. Approximately 20% of these patients are at increased risk of suicide (Suppes et al., 2005). Yet, using only an antidepressant (monotherapy) to treat symptoms of depression increases the risk of treatment-emergent mania. Today, at least, the best course of psychopharmacological management of bipolar disorder appears to be with mood-stabilizing drugs. The clinician may choose to treat with lithium alone or in combination with certain anticonvulsants and/or atypical antipsychotics to maintain euthymia as much as possible.

BDNF is a neurotrophic factor that seems to play a role in a number of psychiatric conditions and illnesses, including depression, mania, schizophrenia, and dementia. In the case of mania/bipolar disorder its role is far less defined than it is in depression. However, there does seem to be some genetic predisposition toward early onset, and toward rapid-cycling bipolar patients who have one particular phenotype of the promoter protein for BDNF, ProBDNF. Interestingly, individuals with the one phenotype (Val66Met or Met66Met) of the gene may be more susceptible to cognitive disorders, such as Alzheimer's and perhaps schizophrenia, and those with the more common phenotype (Val66Val) may be more susceptible to early onset or rapid-cycling bipolar disorder. From an evolutionary standpoint, which is the preferred gene to pass on to future generations? Perhaps this is similar to the situation where people who live in Africa develop genes that offer protection against malaria but that put the carriers at risk for sickle-cell anemia. This research is still in its infancy. Although it does not seem likely that drugs acting via BDNF are clinically relevant today, they will probably become important in the future.

REVIEW QUESTIONS

1. What may be the biggest clinical danger of treating a bipolar patient with an SSRI such as fluoxetine (Prozac) in the absence of a mood stabilizer?
   a. Poor efficacy in relieving depressive symptoms when SSRIs are used as monotherapy
   b. Increases the risk of suicidal thoughts
   c. May trigger a rapid switch in polarity. Patients go rapidly from depressed to manic.
   d. Since the mood stabilizer (e.g., lithium) is needed to increase BDNF, onset of action is slower than when the second drug is included.

2. Harriet Brinkmann is a 22-year-old patient who has been diagnosed as bipolar II for at least 5 years. Which of the following is least likely to be used as a mood-stabilizer?
   a. Alprazolam (Xanax)
   b. Lithium carbonate (Lithobid)
   c. Valproic acid (Depakote)
   d. Quetiapine (Seroquel)

3. Although there are two forms (genotypes) of the gene coding for BDNF, the actual BDNF molecule released by the hippocampus is identical for both genotypes. How then can particular BDNF variants be associated with certain mental illnesses, including bipolar disorder?
   a. The combination of the gene and a particular environment interact (nature plus nurture).
   b. The part of the protein that is altered, although not part of the final BDNF molecule, can alter BDNF release by neurons.
   c. The premise of this argument is false. Since the gene does not affect the final protein (BDNF), it cannot affect the outcome (i.e., mental health vs. mental illness).
   d. When BDNF variants are cleaved, the cleaved-off portions are identical.

4. Which of the following treatments for depression has not been shown to increase BDNF expression and increase neurogenesis in the hippocampus?
   a. Lithium
   b. Sertraline (Zoloft)
   c. Amitriptyline (Elavil)
   d. Electroconvulsive therapy
   e. All of the above have these actions.

5. Johnny Applecore is a patient who, since his mid-teens, has experienced several episodes of persistently unstable mood, involving many periods of mild depression and mild and enjoyable elation. According to Johnny, his moods are totally unrelated to life events. Johnny has never been hospitalized for any psychiatric disorder. Which of the following diagnoses and treatments would be most appropriate for Johnny?
   a. Euthymia—fluoxetine (Prozac) + lithium (Eskalith, Lithobid)
   b. Bipolar I—lithium (Eskalith, Lithobid) only
   c. Bipolar II—venlafaxine extended release (Effexor XR)
   d. Cyclothymia—quetiapine (Seroquel) + escitalopram (Lexapro)

6. It has been hypothesized that a deficiency of BDNF in certain structures in the brain may account for many symptoms of depression and that restoring the levels of BDNF may be the basis for the clinical action of drugs used to treat mood disorders. Of the choices below, which correctly pairs a brain structure involved in mood disorders with the brain region in which it is located?
   a. Hypothalamus—Brainstem
   b. Hippocampus—Limbic system
   c. Frontal lobe(s)—Diencephalon
   d. Medulla oblongata—Brainstem

7. Today, many depressed patients are treated with the extended-release version of venlafaxine (Effexor XR) rather than the instant-release formulation of the drug (Effexor). What are two reasons that this has occurred?
   a. Lower cost and greater efficacy
   b. Lower dose and reduced plasma protein binding

   c. Extended release formulation only affects the CYP2D6 form of cytochrome P450 and is not associated with increased risk of suicide.
   d. Improved compliance and fewer adverse effects

8. With the advent of SSRIs (e.g., fluoxetine) and dual-mechanism drugs (e.g., mirtazapine), what remains the major roadblock to treatment of major depressive disorders?
   a. Slow onset of action (days to weeks)
   b. Extremely low therapeutic indices (e.g., 1–2)
   c. None of these drugs are agonists at the dopamine (D_2) receptor, whose function is most clearly associated with depression.
   d. No antidepressant currently available has been shown to affect brain-derived neurotrophic factor (BDNF).

9. When hospitalization is needed, how do bipolar I and bipolar II patients differ (if at all)?
   a. For bipolar I patients, it is primarily for severe depression.
   b. For bipolar I patients, it is primarily for severe, acute manic symptoms.
   c. For bipolar II patients, it is for severe euthymia.
   d. Since bipolar II is a more severe form of bipolar I, patients with it are hospitalized far more frequently (for mixed episodes).

10. What is oldest mood stabilizer available today in the United States?
    a. Lithium carbonate (Lithobid)
    b. Clozapine (Clozaril)
    c. Olanzapine (Zyprexa)
    d. Carbamazepine (Tegretol)

REFERENCES

Ali, S., & Milev, R. (2003). Switch to mania upon discontinuation of antidepressants in patients with mood disorders: A review of the literature. *Canadian Journal of Psychiatry—Revue Canadienne De Psychiatrie, 48*(4), 258–264.

American Psychiatric Association. (2000). *Diagnostic and statistical manual of mental disorders: DSM-IV.* (4th ed.) Washington, DC: American Psychiatric Association.

Bueller, J. A., Aftab, M., Sen, S., Gomez-Hassan, D., Burmeister, M., & Zubieta, J. K. (2006). BDNF Val66Met allele is associated with reduced hippocampal volume in healthy subjects. *Biological Psychiatry, 59*(9), 812–815.

Cade, J. F. (1949). Lithium salts in the treatment of psychotic excitement. *Medical Journal of Australia, 2*(10), 349–352.

Calabrese, J. R., Huffman, R. F., White, R. L., Edwards, S., Thompson, T. R., Ascher, J. A., et al. (2008). Lamotrigine in the acute treatment of bipolar depression: Results of five double-blind, placebo-controlled clinical trials. *Bipolar Disorders, 10*(2), 323–333.

Calabrese, J. R., Keck, P. E., Jr., Macfadden, W., Minkwitz, M., Ketter, T. A., Weisler, R. H., et al. (2005). A randomized, double-blind, placebo-controlled trial of quetiapine in the treatment of bipolar I or II depression. *American Journal of Psychiatry, 162*(7), 1351–1360.

Deeks, E. D., & Keating, G. M. (2008). Spotlight on olanzapine/fluoxetine in acute bipolar depression. *CNS Drugs, 22*(9), 793–795.

Duman, R. S., Nakagawa, S., & Malberg, J. (2001). Regulation of adult neurogenesis by antidepressant treatment. *Neuropsychopharmacology, 25*(6), 836–844.

Dunlop, B. W., & Nemeroff, C. B. (2007). The role of dopamine in the pathophysiology of depression.[see comment]. *Archives of General Psychiatry, 64*(3), 327–337.

Egan, M. F., Kojima, M., Callicott, J. H., Goldberg, T. E., Kolachana, B. S., Bertolino, A., et al. (2003). The BDNF val66met polymorphism affects activity-dependent secretion of BDNF and human memory and hippocampal function. *Cell, 112*(2), 257–269.

Fan, J., & Sklar, P. (2008). Genetics of bipolar disorder: Focus on BDNF Val66Met polymorphism. *Novartis Foundation Symposium, 289,* 60–72.

Foland, L. C., Altshuler, L. L., Sugar, C. A., Lee, A. D., Leow, A. D., Townsend, J., et al. (2008). Increased volume of the amygdala and hippocampus in bipolar patients treated with lithium. *Neuroreport, 19*(2), 221–224.

Freeman, M. P., & Freeman, S. A. (2006). Lithium: Clinical considerations in internal medicine. *American Journal of Medicine, 119*(6), 478–481.

Fukumoto, T., Morinobu, S., Okamoto, Y., Kagaya, A., & Yamawaki, S. (2001). Chronic lithium treatment increases the expression of brain-derived neurotrophic factor in the rat brain. *Psychopharmacology, 158*(1), 100–106.

Gajwani, P., Forsthoff, A., Muzina, D., Amann, B., Gao, K., Elhaj, O., et al. (2005). Antiepileptic drugs in mood-disordered patients. *Epilepsia, 46*(Suppl 4), 38–44.

Gajwani, P., Kemp, D. E., Muzina, D. J., Xia, G., Gao, K., & Calabrese, J. R. (2006). Acute treatment of mania: An update on new medications. *Current Psychiatry Reports, 8*(6), 504–509.

Geller, B., Badner, J. A., Tillman, R., Christian, S. L., Bolhofner, K., & Cook, E. H., Jr. (2004). Linkage disequilibrium of the brain-derived neurotrophic factor Val66Met polymorphism in children with a prepubertal and early adolescent bipolar disorder phenotype. *American Journal of Psychiatry, 161*(9), 1698–1700.

Goldberg, J. F., & Citrome, L. (2005). Latest therapies for bipolar disorder looking beyond lithium. *Postgraduate Medicine, 117*(2), 25–26.

Goodwin, F. K., & Jamison, K. R. (1990). *Manic-depressive illness.* New York: Oxford University Press.

Green, E. K., Raybould, R., Macgregor, S., Hyde, S., Young, A. H., O'Donovan, M. C., et al. (2006). Genetic variation of brain-derived neurotrophic factor (BDNF) in bipolar disorder: Case-control study of over 3000 individuals from the UK. *British Journal of Psychiatry, 188,* 21–25.

Grunze, H. (2005). Reevaluating therapies for bipolar depression. *Journal of Clinical Psychiatry, 66*(Suppl 5), 17–25.

Hariri, A. R., Goldberg, T. E., Mattay, V. S., Kolachana, B. S., Callicott, J. H., Egan, M. F., et al. (2003). Brain-derived neurotrophic factor val66met polymorphism affects human memory-related hippocampal activity and predicts memory performance. *Journal of Neuroscience, 23*(17), 6690–6694.

Healy, D., Harris, M., Farquhar, F., Tschinkel, S., & Le Noury, J. (2008). Historical overview: Kraepelin's impact on psychiatry. *European Archives of Psychiatry & Clinical Neuroscience, 258*(Suppl 2), 18–24.

Hong, C. J., Yu, Y. W., Lin, C. H., & Tsai, S. J. (2003). An association study of a brain-derived neurotrophic factor Val66Met polymorphism and clozapine response of schizophrenic patients. *Neuroscience Letters, 349*(3), 206–208.

Introduction: Primer on molecular genetics. Human Genome Program, U.S. Department of Energy, Primer on Molecular Genetics, Washington, DC, 1992. http://www.ornl.gov/sci/techresources/Human_Genome/publicat/primer/prim1.html

Kessler, R. C., Akiskal, H. S., Angst, J., Guyer, M., Hirschfeld, R. M., Merikangas, K. R., et al. (2006). Validity of the assessment of bipolar spectrum disorders in the WHO CIDI 3.0. *Journal of Affective Disorders, 96*(3), 259–269.

Kunugi, H., Iijima, Y., Tatsumi, M., Yoshida, M., Hashimoto, R., Kato, T., et al. (2004). No association between the Val66Met polymorphism of the brain-derived neurotrophic factor gene and bipolar disorder in a Japanese population: A multicenter study. *Biological Psychiatry, 56*(5), 376–378.

Lohoff, F. W., Sander, T., Ferraro, T. N., Dahl, J. P., Gallinat, J., & Berrettini, W. H. (2005). Confirmation of association between the Val66Met polymorphism in the brain-derived neurotrophic factor (BDNF) gene and bipolar I disorder. *American Journal of Medical Genetics. Part B, Neuropsychiatric Genetics: The Official Publication of the International Society of Psychiatric Genetics, 139*(1), 51–53.

McNamara, J. O. (2006). Chapter 19: Pharmacotherapies of the Epilepsies. In L. L. Brunton, J. S. Lazo, & K. L. Parker (Eds.), *Goodman & Gilman's the pharmacological basis of therapeutics* (11th ed.). New York: McGraw-Hill.

Moore, G. J., Bebchuk, J. M., Wilds, I. B., Chen, G., & Manji, H. K. (2000). Lithium-induced increase in human brain grey matter. *Lancet, 356*(9237), 1241–1242.

Moreno, C., Laje, G., Blanco, C., Jiang, H., Schmidt, A. B., & Olfson, M. (2007). National trends in the outpatient diagnosis and treatment of bipolar disorder in youth. *Archives of General Psychiatry, 64*(9), 1032–1039.

Nakata, K., Ujike, H., Sakai, A., Uchida, N., Nomura, A., Imamura, T., et al. (2003). Association study of the brain-derived neurotrophic factor (BDNF) gene with bipolar disorder. *Neuroscience Letters, 337*(1), 17–20.

Neves-Pereira, M., Cheung, J. K., Pasdar, A., Zhang, F., Breen, G., Yates, P., et al. (2005). BDNF gene is a risk factor for schizophrenia in a Scottish population. *Molecular Psychiatry, 10*(2), 208–212.

Neves-Pereira, M., Mundo, E., Muglia, P., King, N., Macciardi, F., & Kennedy, J. L. (2002). The brain-derived neurotrophic factor gene confers susceptibility to bipolar disorder: Evidence from a family-based association study. *American Journal of Human Genetics, 71*(3), 651–655.

Ohgami, H., Terao, T., Shiotsuki, I., Ishii, N., & Iwata, N. (2009). Lithium levels in drinking water and risk of suicide. *British Journal of Psychiatry, 194*(5), 464–465.

Perris, C. (1990). The importance of Karl Leonhard's classification of endogenous psychoses. *Psychopathology, 23*(4–6), 282–290.

Post, R. M. (2007). Role of BDNF in bipolar and unipolar disorder: Clinical and theoretical implications. *Journal of Psychiatric Research, 41*(12), 979–990.

Seidah, N. G., Benjannet, S., Pareek, S., Chretien, M., & Murphy, R. A. (1996). Cellular processing of the neurotrophin precursors of NT3 and BDNF by the mammalian proprotein convertases. *FEBS Letters, 379*(3), 247–250.

Shaltiel, G., Chen, G., & Manji, H. K. (2007). Neurotrophic signaling cascades in the pathophysiology and treatment of bipolar disorder. *Current Opinion in Pharmacology, 7*(1), 22–26.

Skibinska, M., Hauser, J., Czerski, P. M., Leszczynska-Rodziewicz, A., Kosmowska, M., Kapelski, P., et al. (2004). Association analysis of brain-derived neurotrophic factor (BDNF) gene

Val66Met polymorphism in schizophrenia and bipolar affective disorder. *World Journal of Biological Psychiatry, 5*(4), 215–220.

Sklar, P., Gabriel, S. B., McInnis, M. G., Bennett, P., Lim, Y. M., Tsan, G., et al. (2002). Family-based association study of 76 candidate genes in bipolar disorder: BDNF is a potential risk locus: . . . . Brain-derived neutrophic factor. *Molecular Psychiatry, 7*(6), 579–593.

Suppes, T., Kelly, D. I., & Perla, J. M. (2005). Challenges in the management of bipolar depression. *Journal of Clinical Psychiatry, 66*(Suppl 5), 11–16.

Watson, S., & Young, A. H. (2001). The place of lithium salts in psychiatric practice 50 years on. *Current Opinion in Psychiatry, 14*(1), 57–63.

Wehr, T. A., & Goodwin, F. K. (1979). Rapid cycling in manic-depressives induced by tricyclic antidepressants. *Archives of General Psychiatry, 36*(5), 555–559.

WHO (2001). *Burden of mental and behavioural disorders (Chapter 2).* Retrieved 5/2/2009, 2009, from http://www.who.int/whr/2001/chapter2/en/index3.html

CHAPTER 4

Antipsychotic Pharmacotherapy

"I do not suffer from insanity, I enjoy every minute of it."

EDGAR ALLAN POE

"If you talk to God, you are praying; if God talks to you, you have schizophrenia."

THOMAS SZASZ

GETTING PERSONAL*

I fell in love when I was 17 and over the next four years that relationship slowly disintegrated as schizophrenia took over my life. I lost interest in school. I actually scored in the top three percentile in a province wide Mathematics contest in Grade 11, and never finished another mathematics or physics course again. At university I experienced a lot of emotional turmoil and was incapable and uninterested in long-term romantic relationships. I was also incapable of planning my future, of choosing a career path, and applied to graduate school because I had so much trouble getting work of any sort. . . .

Within two years I had relapsed and was homeless on the streets of Calgary. I was sleeping in the single men's hostel and weak from hunger. I didn't get to eat anything at all for over a week because I had no money. I was being watched and followed by this World War II character who demanded

*From *The Experience of Schizophrenia* by Ian Chovil. http://www.chovil.com/story2.html. Retrieved 22 October 2006. *Used with the permission of author.*

I get a job in construction and shape up. Tibetan Buddhists were reading my mind everywhere I went in Calgary because I had caused the Mt. St. Helen's eruption earlier that year. They were training me to become a great Buddhist saint which required a life of abject poverty and isolation. I went for ten years more or less like that, completely alone, living five years out west and five years in Toronto, marginally employed, homeless for periods, with no friends, no lovers. At first I was going to be a Tibetan saint, then I realized I was a pawn in a secret war that would determine the fate of humanity, then I was the chosen one that the aliens would rescue from the earth before the great nuclear war. I was having a lot of trouble taking care of myself because I was experiencing a lot of reality distortion and disorganization, prominent symptoms of schizophrenia.

I had imaginary friends and powerful enemies and I got a lot of messages and was in constant telepathic contact with someone most of the last five years. I discovered antigravity and understood human evolution and my imaginary wife and I were going to become an aliens and have eternal life traveling to the end of time where all matter had turned into energy and all that remained was music and space. I knew I was going to become an alien in 1991 because I saw a book written by Nostradamus entitled 3791. I turned 37 in 1991 so that was obviously his message to me from the 1500s. I was living in a cockroach-infested illegal rooming house and changing light bulbs as they burned out in the Hudson's Bay department store, afraid of my enemies who wanted to take my place as the most important man in human history.

A number of things happened. I got in trouble with the law, as happens fairly often in untreated schizophrenia, I became alcoholic, which also happens fairly often with untreated schizophrenia, and I lost my job. I had convinced the aliens to transfer my mind to another body, an easy thing for them, and a statement of how miserable my life was at the time. When I woke up, still in my body, I became furious, and started breaking windows in the rooming house. Someone called the police who interrupted my rampage and I spent a couple of nights in jail. Actually one night in a holding cell, a day in court, a night in the Don Jail, another day in court and I was free. . . .

My behavior became increasingly bizarre as my drinking progressed, and I was fired from my job. At first this was great. The aliens obviously had listened to me and I was going to win the Provincial lottery, at least $10 million and have a vacation. I didn't win though and my income went from $11 an hour to Unemployment Insurance, to Welfare. By the end I was brewing my own beer in plastic pails unable to quit drinking. I was eating at the Scott Mission to afford the ingredients and missing rent payments. I could see the men sleeping on hot air vents nearby and knew that that was where I was heading. The aliens controlled everything that happened to me and I made one last attempt to argue against them.

By that time my probation was almost over and the psychiatrists were suggesting I become a patient at a psychiatric hospital for alcoholism, and I agreed to go. I had to wait something like six months before there was a bed for me. As I sobered up my delusions, or at least my faith in their validity faded and I started on antipsychotics and took up residence in Guelph, still unconvinced I had schizophrenia. The next three years or so I was very unhappy slowly coming to an awareness that I had schizophrenia and aliens weren't going to rescue me.

My mood slowly came around, I made a few friends, eventually tried some volunteer work, and then some paid work. Each year has seen an improvement in the quality of my life. Each year I have been able to be a little more productive, a little more comfortable with people, a little less anxious. I've tried a lot of things and quit a lot of things. I've had to manage my symptoms and illness, trying to balance my life, budgeting for essentials and desires. I spent most of the last nine years counting my pennies but lately I have been quite comfortable.

INTRODUCTION

Descriptions of what is now referred to as schizophrenia date back to the days of Egyptian hieroglyphics. The modern notion of this illness, however, dates back to nineteenth-century Europe. Although the German psychiatrist Emil Kraepelin is generally credited for introducing *dementia praecox* (premature dementia) as a distinct diagnostic entity in his *Lehrbuch der Psychiatrie* (1893), the first published use of this term was by the French physician Benedict-Augustin Morel (1852–1853). What Kraepelin famously did was to split the established unitary model of psychosis into two distinct forms: manic depression and dementia praecox. Kraepelin was also a colleague and research partner of Alois Alzheimer, and a codiscoverer of Alzheimer's disease. In fact, it was Kraepelin's laboratory that discovered the pathologic basis of this disorder.

Eugen Bleuler (1908) introduced the term *schizophrenia* (from the Greek for "splitting of the mind") as an alternative to dementia praecox. Bleuler correctly noted in his seminal publication, *Dementia Praecox oder Gruppe der Schizophrenien* (1911), that the disorder did not necessarily include dementia nor did it always manifest in youth. Rather, it was characterized by the fragmented thinking of the patients.

Imagine being a mental health practitioner in 1949. A patient comes in with clear signs of schizophrenia, including paranoid delusions, auditory hallucinations, flat affect, avolition, impaired memory, and impaired executive function. What is the best way to treat this patient? Perhaps the psychotherapeutic methods of Sigmund Freud could be used to help the patient identify the underlying root cause(s) of the disorder. Would prescribing risperidone (Risperdal) or haloperidol (Haldol) be an option? Unfortunately, these drugs haven't been discovered yet. Would a little electroconvulsive therapy or perhaps a lobotomy help? Maybe the patient will be put into a sanitarium to rest and talk and possibly recover (or at the least not embarrass the family). In the middle of the twentieth century clinicians had limited treatment options and effective drug therapy was not yet available, leaving patients and their families with few choices for dealing with this debilitating mental illness.

Meanwhile, in France in 1952, Henri Laborit was looking for an effective preanesthetic medication, when he tried chlorpromazine (Thorazine), which was unsuccessfully developed as an antihistamine (Lopez-Munoz et al., 2005), to help calm his patients. Although it was calming, it also lowered patients' blood pressure (by blocking alpha-1 receptors) far too much to be clinically useful. However, Laborit hypothesized that chlorpromazine might be useful for calming psychiatric patients. When it was given to patients with diverse psychiatric problems, not only did it have a quieting effect, it also improved many symptoms in schizophrenic patients, much more so than other tranquilizers (Whitaker, 2003). Thus was born the age of biological psychiatry. In this new age, mental illness was finally accepted as having a biologic basis, the result of a specific chemical imbalance(s) in the brain. With this new understanding, drugs could now be used to potentially correct the problem . . . or create it.

In the 1950s and 1960s, numerous experiments were carried out with drugs to produce a controlled, predictable, and reversible clinical model of schizophrenia in order to develop more effective treatments for this disorder. All of this was helped along by a serendipitous laboratory accident at Sandoz Laboratories in Basel, Switzerland, in 1943. Albert Hofmann, a well-respected researcher, was studying derivatives of ergot alkaloids (products produced by grain fungus) to find a better labor-inducing drug, and to see if these compounds had any other unique or useful pharmacological properties. The 25th chemical in the samples he looked at was innocuously named in German *lysergsäure-diethylamid* (LSD). In the course of his studies, on that fateful day, he may have "accidentally" ingested a minute amount of the drug before bicycling home from work. Here is his account of the next few hours:

> Last Friday, April 16, 1943, I was forced to interrupt my work in the laboratory in the middle of the afternoon and proceed home, being affected by a remarkable restlessness, combined with a slight dizziness. At home I lay down and sank into a not unpleasant intoxicated-like condition, characterized by an extremely stimulated imagination. In a dreamlike state, with eyes closed (I found the daylight to be unpleasantly glaring), I perceived an uninterrupted stream of fantastic pictures, extraordinary shapes with intense, kaleidoscopic play of colors. After some two hours this condition faded away. (Hofmann, 1980)

Three days later, pretty sure of the chemical he had accidentally absorbed in his lab, Hofmann conducted an experiment in which he took 250-microgram (0.25 mg) of LSD-25. What happened next is well worth reading.

> By now it was already clear to me that LSD had been the cause of the remarkable experience of the previous Friday, for the altered perceptions were of the same type as before, only much more intense. I had to struggle to speak intelligibly. I asked my laboratory assistant, who was informed of the self-experiment, to escort me home. We went by bicycle, no automobile being available because of wartime restrictions on their use. On the way home, my condition began to assume threatening forms. Everything in my field of vision wavered and was distorted as if seen in a curved mirror. I also had the sensation of being unable to move from the spot. Nevertheless, my assistant later told me that we had traveled very rapidly. Finally, we arrived at home safe and sound, and I was just barely capable of asking my companion to summon our family doctor and request milk from the neighbors.
>
> In spite of my delirious, bewildered condition, I had brief periods of clear and effective thinking—and chose milk as a nonspecific antidote for poisoning.
>
> The dizziness and sensation of fainting became so strong at times that I could no longer hold myself erect, and had to lie down on a sofa. My surroundings had now transformed themselves in more terrifying ways. Everything in the room spun around, and the familiar objects and pieces of furniture assumed grotesque, threatening forms. They were in continuous motion, animated, as if driven by an inner restlessness. The lady next door, whom I scarcely recognized, brought me milk—in the course of the evening I drank more than two liters. She was no longer Mrs. R., but rather a malevolent, insidious witch with a colored mask.
>
> Even worse than these demonic transformations of the outer world, were the alterations that I perceived in myself, in my inner being. Every exertion of my will, every attempt to put an end to the disintegration of the outer world and the dissolution of my ego, seemed to be wasted effort. A demon had invaded me, had taken possession of my body, mind, and soul. I jumped up and screamed, trying to free myself from him, but then sank down again and lay helpless on the sofa. The substance, with which I had wanted to experiment, had vanquished me. It was the demon that scornfully triumphed over my will. I was seized by the dreadful fear of going insane. I was taken to another world, another place, another time. My body seemed to be without sensation, lifeless, strange. Was I dying? Was this the transition? At times I believed

myself to be outside my body, and then perceived clearly, as an outside observer, the complete tragedy of my situation. I had not even taken leave of my family (my wife, with our three children had traveled that day to visit her parents, in Lucerne). Would they ever understand that I had not experimented thoughtlessly, irresponsibly, but rather with the utmost caution, and that such a result was in no way foreseeable? My fear and despair intensified, not only because a young family should lose its father, but also because I dreaded leaving my chemical research work, which meant so much to me, unfinished in the midst of fruitful, promising development. Another reflection took shape, an idea full of bitter irony: if I was now forced to leave this world prematurely, it was because of this lysergic acid diethylamide that I myself had brought forth into the world.

By the time the doctor arrived, the climax of my despondent condition had already passed. My laboratory assistant informed him about my self-experiment, as I myself was not yet able to formulate a coherent sentence. He shook his head in perplexity, after my attempts to describe the mortal danger that threatened my body. He could detect no abnormal symptoms other than extremely dilated pupils. Pulse, blood pressure, breathing were all normal. He saw no reason to prescribe any medication. Instead he conveyed me to my bed and stood watch over me. Slowly I came back from a weird, unfamiliar world to reassuring everyday reality. The horror softened and gave way to a feeling of good fortune and gratitude, the more normal perceptions and thoughts returned, and I became more confident that the danger of insanity was conclusively past.

Now, little by little I could begin to enjoy the unprecedented colors and plays of shapes that persisted behind my closed eyes. Kaleidoscopic, fantastic images surged in on me, alternating, variegated, opening and then closing themselves in circles and spirals, exploding in colored fountains, rearranging and hybridizing themselves in constant flux. It was particularly remarkable how every acoustic perception, such as the sound of a door handle or a passing automobile, became transformed into optical perceptions. Every sound generated a vividly changing image, with its own consistent form and color.

Thus was born the first truly bad acid trip. Several years after the clinical trail, Sandoz made the drug available for clinical use. Dr. Hofmann's trial dose of 0.25 mg was 10 times higher than the "recommended" clinical dose. The drug is so potent that 1 gram—the weight of a paper clip—is enough to send 10,000 to 20,000 people on a 12-hour LSD trip. After documenting his LSD experiences, Hofmann returned to his research. He died on April 29, 2008, at the age of 102.

The indications and dosage recommended for the use of this drug, now officially named Delysid (between 1947 and the mid 1960s, when it was removed from the market), by Sandoz Pharmaceuticals (Hofmann, 1980) were as follows:

(a) Analytical psychotherapy, to elicit release of repressed material and provide mental relaxation, particularly in anxiety states and obsessional neuroses.

The initial dose is 25 mcg (1/4 of an ampoule or 1 tablet). This dose is increased at each treatment by 25 mcg until the optimum dose (usually between 50 and 200 mcg) is found. The individual treatments are best given at intervals of one week.

(b) Experimental studies on the nature of psychoses: By taking Delysid himself, the psychiatrist is able to gain an insight into the world of ideas and sensations of mental patients. Delysid can also be used to induce model psychoses of short duration in normal subjects, thus facilitating studies on the pathogenesis of mental disease.

In normal subjects, doses of 25 to 75 mcg re generally sufficient to produce a hallucinatory psychosis (on an average 1 mcg/kg body weight). In certain forms of psychosis and in chronic alcoholism, higher doses are necessary (2 to 4 mcg/kg body weight).

Reread item *b* and then try to recall the last time a pharmaceutical company recommended that prescribers take a drug in order to understand what their patients experience. Despite his best intentions, Hofmann was both right and wrong in his ideas. He was right that certain drugs can mimic the symptoms of schizophrenia, but he was wrong in the drug he chose to model the illness. There are two important differences between the altered state of mind produced by LSD and that psychotic state of the schizophrenic patient. First, LSD-induced hallucinations are for the most part visual whereas a hallmark symptom of schizophrenia is auditory hallucinations. Second, with LSD, users are aware that they are in a hallucinogenic state, but with schizophrenia, the patient is unaware.

In the decades since the pioneering work of the 1950s and 1960s, a host of drugs have been developed to treat schizophrenia. Although they vary chemically, they all have certain common features (Baldessarini & Tarazi, 2006). They all reduce the positive symptoms of schizophrenia, which include:

- Delusions
- Hallucinations
- Disorganized speech/thinking
- Grossly disorganized behavior
- Catatonic behaviors

Until recently, these drugs also shared common neurochemical action: they all blocked dopamine (DA) receptors. In fact, the degree to which they blocked the D_2 subtype of the receptor was highly correlated with their clinical efficacy. Unfortunately, this first generation of antipsychotic drugs (FGAs) shared a common but serious adverse effect; to one degree or another they all produced movement disorders, ranging from dystonia, to dyskinesia, to pseudoparkinsonism (extrapyramidal symptoms, EPS).

Since all the early clinically available antipsychotics had the same neurochemical action (blocking D_2 receptors), most investigators concluded that schizophrenia is primarily a mental illness that results from excess in dopamine activity somewhere in the brain—the so-called Dopamine Hypothesis of Schizophrenia, now in its third major iteration (Howes & Kapur, 2009). If this hypothesis is true, then where is this excess occurring? There are some clues that can help identify the location.

NEUROANATOMY AND NEUROPHYSIOLOGY

In the brain, there are four pathways in which DA is the neurotransmitter (Figure 4-1) (Nestler, Hyman, & Malenka, 2008; Stahl, 2008). These are the mesolimbic (ML), mesocortical (MC), nigrostriatal (NS), and tuberoinfundibular (TI) pathways.

MESOLIMBIC PATHWAY (ML)

The mesolimbic pathway begins at the ventral portion of the tegmentum in the midbrain and runs to the nucleus accumbens in the limbic system. This is believed to be the area of the brain that mediates the positive symptoms of schizophrenia (Stahl, 2008). Drugs and diseases that increase DA here

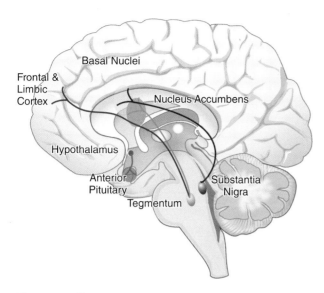

Nigrostriatal (Substantia Nigra to Basal Nuclei)
Mesolimbic (Ventral Tegmentum to Nucleus Accumbens)
Mesocortical (Ventral Tegmentum to Frontal and Limbic Cortex)
Tuberoinfundibular (Hypothalamus to Anterior Pituitary)

FIGURE 4-1 Four key dopamine pathways: mesolimbic, mesocortical, nigrostriatal, and tuberoinfundibular.

increase positive symptoms, whereas drugs that block DA receptors (particularly the D_2 subtype) decrease these symptoms. Other than schizophrenia, positive signs of schizophrenia can be mimicked by high, repeated doses of two common drugs of abuse—amphetamines and cocaine—both of which can cause symptoms indistinguishable from paranoid schizophrenia. Antipsychotic drugs block this receptor and reduce the positive symptoms of schizophrenia (and amphetamine psychosis.) These findings, according to Stahl (2008), allow for the refinement of the DA Hypothesis of Schizophrenia to the Mesolimbic DA Hypothesis for the Positive Symptoms of Schizophrenia.

MESOCORTICAL PATHWAY (MC)

The mesocortical pathway also begins at the ventral portion of the tegmentum but it goes to the frontal and limbic cortex. It is believed that DA in these pathways plays a role in mediating the negative (and possibly the cognitive) symptoms of schizophrenia.

Negative symptoms of schizophrenia include:

- Lack of emotion—the inability to enjoy regular activities
- Low energy—the person tends to sit around and sleep much more than normal
- Lack of interest in life, low motivation
- Affective flattening—a blank, non-expressive or blunted facial expression or less lively facial movements, flat voice (lack of normal intonations and variance)
- Alogia (difficulty or inability to speak)
- Inappropriate social skills or lack of interest or ability to socialize with other people
- Inability to make friends or keep friends, or not caring to have friends

- Social isolation—person spends most of the day alone or only with close family

Cognitive symptoms of schizophrenia include:

- Disorganized thinking
- Slow thinking
- Difficulty understanding
- Poor concentration
- Poor memory
- Difficulty expressing thoughts
- Difficulty integrating thoughts, feelings, and behavior

Interestingly, research suggests that these symptoms are actually due to a deficit (not a surplus) in DA levels or underactivity in this pathway. Although the deficit might be primary, it is more likely that it is a secondary response to an excess of 5-HT that inhibits DA release. This inverse relationship between DA activity and negative symptoms (i.e., lower activity leads to more symptoms) in the MC pathway might explain why these symptoms do not always improve, and might actually worsen with antipsychotics that act solely by blocking DA receptors. However, it also may help explain why the newer second-generation antipsychotics, which have action mediated by 5-HT, may be better than the older drugs (which only block DA receptors) at alleviating the negative symptoms of schizophrenia.

NIGROSTRIATAL PATHWAY (NS)

The nigrostriatal pathway begins at the substantia nigra in the midbrain and terminates at the basal nuclei, which includes the striatum (caudate nucleus plus putamen) and the globus pallidus. This area of the brain helps regulate posture and voluntary movement. Coming into the striatum (Figure 4-2) are excitatory (+) ACh and GLU neurons and inhibitory (−) DA neurons. When these opposing pathways are "balanced," motor function is normal. When they are out of balance, abnormal motor (neurological) symptoms occur.

In Parkinson's disease, the substantia nigra degenerates and the patient develops a characteristic set of movement difficulties (resting tremor, akinesia, and rigidity). Elevated activity, due to excess transmitter or receptor super-sensitivity, may also produce motor problems for the patient, including choreas, dyskinesia, and tics.

When traditional (first generation) antipsychotics are used to treat schizophrenia, they also block the DA receptors in this pathway, resulting in a Parkinsonism-like syndrome (extrapyramidal symptoms, EPS). Stahl (2008) describes these neurological symptoms of treatment as "the cost of doing business." Up until the last decade or so, the more clinically effective the antipsychotic, the more likely it was to produce EPS. Newer drugs are far less likely to produce these symptoms and are now often the drugs of choice for treating psychoses.

TUBEROINFUNDIBULAR PATHWAY (TI)

The tuberoinfundibular pathway begins at the hypothalamus and goes just a short distance to the anterior pituitary gland. Normally DA inhibits prolactin release by the pituitary. Prolactin is a hormone that prepares the breasts for lactation in women, but the hormone's function in men is not well understood. When drugs or disease affect this pathway female patients may experience galactorrhea, amenorrhea, and sexual dysfunction.

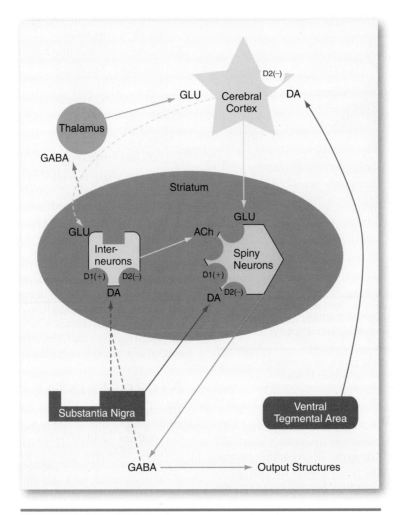

FIGURE 4-2 Dopaminergic (DA), cholinergic (ACh), and glutamatergic (GLU) influence on the striatum. GABA coming from the striatum mediates normal motor function. The amount of GABA released from striatal spiny neurons depends on the balance of GLU excitatory input from the cerebral cortex and ACh from interneurons and inhibitory DA input from the substantia nigra. Blockage of DA neurons from the substantia nigra leads to Parkinson-like symptoms in patients taking first-generation antipsychotics.

ANTIPSYCHOTICS

From the 1960s through the 1980s, a wide range of clinically useful antipsychotics became available. They all appeared to work by blocking D_2 receptors in the limbic system but all produced, to a varying degree, a number of adverse effects because they nonselectively blocked DA receptors throughout the brain, rather than in the area(s) of the brain believed to be disturbed in schizophrenia. Besides neurological adverse effects, other problems are common with these drugs because they also affect many neurotransmitter systems including muscarinic, adrenergic, and histaminergic receptors (Table 4-1).

TABLE 4-1 Other Adverse Effects of FGAs

SYMPTOMS	RECEPTOR BLOCKED
Dry mouth, blurred vision, racing heart, constipation, drowsiness	Muscarinic cholinergic
Weight gain, drowsiness	H1-histaminergic
↓ BP, dizziness, drowsiness	α_1-adrenergic

Beginning in the 1990s significant changes in treatment occurred. In 1990 clozapine (Clozaril) was approved in the United States after a large clinical trial proved its superiority over conventional or first-generation antipsychotics (FGA) (Lieberman, Golden, Stroup, & McEvoy, 2000). Not only did it work better in controlling both positive and negative symptoms of schizophrenia, it did not produce extrapyramidal symptoms. Because of potentially life-threatening adverse effects, however, clozapine is currently not a drug of first choice in treating schizophrenia. But it led to the development of risperidone and other "atypical" or second-generation antipsychotics (SGA). The terms *atypical* and *SGA* are often applied interchangeably to newer antipsychotics that relieve the symptoms of schizophrenia but do not produce EPS (or at least do so to a degree far less than FGAs) (Table 4-2).

The SGAs differ from the FGAs neurochemically. Not only do SGAs block DA receptors, but they also block 5-HT

receptors (Kinon & Lieberman, 1996). How does blocking a second neurotransmitter improve clinical outcomes and reduce CNS-mediated side effects?

To understand this, it is important to comprehend the relationship between 5-HT and DA neurotransmission in the brain. All four DA pathways in the brain have presynaptic 5-HT_{2A} receptors (Figure 4-3). With autoreceptors, a neurotransmitter (NT) acts on the neuron that released it to inhibit additional release of that same NT (e.g., NE acting on presynaptic α_2 receptors). Serotonin or 5-HT can act in a similar manner on DA-containing neurons. This receptor for 5-HT is a heteroreceptor, one that alters the release of a different NT. Blocking presynaptic 5-HT_{2A} receptors increases the release of DA.

But isn't the goal in treating schizophrenia to decrease excessive DA function, not increase it? How is it possible to get clinical improvement and reduce adverse effects by elevating DA levels? Part of the answer is that the process in Figure 4-3 is overly simplified. The relationship between 5-HT_{2A} presynaptic receptors and DA release is somewhat distinct for each of the four DA pathways. By looking at each pathway in terms of 5-HT_{2A} and DA receptors, the neurochemical actions of FGAs and SGAs, and the clinical and adverse effects of each of these classes of drugs, can be seen.

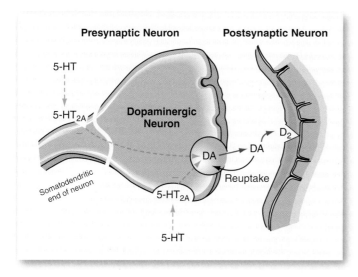

FIGURE 4-3 Influence of 5-HT on dopamine (DA) releasing neurons. 5-HT, acting on 5-HT_{2A} receptors either at the terminal or further back along the dopaminergic neuron (i.e., on a dendrite) can inhibit the release of DA.

ANTIPSYCHOTIC DRUGS AND BRAIN DOPAMINE PATHWAYS

NIGROSTRIATAL PATHWAY

In the NS pathway the relationship between presynaptic 5-HT receptors and DA release is strong and specific: blocking presynaptic 5-HT_{2A} receptors increases DA release (Figure 4-3).

All FGAs are DA-receptor antagonists in the brain, including the areas unrelated to schizophrenia. Because they block the fully functional, undamaged D_2 receptors in the striatum, patients frequently develop EPS. This occurs because the balance between DA and ACh necessary for normal fine

TABLE 4-2 Examples of First-Generation and Second-Generation Antipsychotics

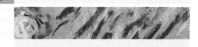

FIRST-GENERATION	SECOND-GENERATION
Chlorpromazine (*Thorazine*)	Clozapine (*Clozaril*)
Fluphenazine (*Prolixin*)	Olanzapine (*Zyprexa*)
Thioridazine (*Mellaril*)	Risperidone (*Risperdal*)
Trifluperazine (*Stelazine*)	Quetiapine (*Seroquel*)
Haloperidol (*Haldol*)	Ziprasidone (*Geodon*)
	Aripiprazole (*Abilify*)

motor function is lost (Figure 4-2). In other words, as cognitive function returns with drug treatment, patients often have to deal with neurologic side effects.

Although SGAs also block the same DA receptors, EPS is far less common. That's because the SGAs have a dual action; they are 5-HT antagonists as well as DA receptor antagonists. Since blocking presynaptic 5-HT$_{2A}$ receptors in the striatum increases the release of DA (Figure 4-3), the imbalance between ACh and DA seen with older drugs is less prominent with the newer drugs and EPS is not seen.

MESOCORTICAL PATHWAY

In the MC pathway, the relationship between 5-HT receptors and DA release is similar to those described for the NS pathway. Again, FGAs block D$_2$ receptors in this location and everywhere else. In fact, blocking the mesocortical D$_2$ receptors actually worsens the negative symptoms of schizophrenia. Thus, while older drugs improve some symptoms of schizophrenia, they may worsen other symptoms.

SGAs, on the other hand, increase DA release via by blocking presynaptic 5-HT$_{2A}$ receptors, as noted above. Interestingly, SGAs are better at antagonizing 5-HT$_{2A}$ than they are at antagonizing D$_2$ receptors (leading to elevated DA levels) in the cortex. Here, it appears that the elevation of DA levels makes these drugs more effective than older drugs in treating both the negative and cognitive symptoms of schizophrenia.

TUBEROINFUNDIBULAR PATHWAY

In addition to the DA input from the hypothalamus, the pituitary gland receives serotonergic input. Whereas DA (acting at D$_2$ receptors) reduces prolactin release, 5-HT has the opposite effect (via 5-HT$_{2A}$ receptors). Conversely, blocking D$_2$ receptors here with FGAs increases prolactin release and is associated with prolactinemia (excess prolactin release). Again, because SGAs block 5-HT$_{2A}$ receptors, this effect is much less likely to be encountered.

MESOLIMBIC PATHWAY

Finally, in the ML pathway, both FGAs and SGAs block D$_2$ receptors and reduce the positive symptoms of schizophrenia. However, since the influence of presynaptic 5-HT$_{2A}$ on DA release is far less prominent in the limbic system than in the other three DA pathways, SGAs do not increase DA release, which would offset the beneficial effects of blocking the D$_2$ receptor.

PUTTING IT TOGETHER: PART I

In summary, FGAs block D$_2$ receptors throughout the brain, which is responsible for both the beneficial and adverse effects of these drugs. Blocking these receptors in the limbic system reduces the positive symptoms of schizophrenia. However, blocking the remaining DA pathways is responsible for most of their adverse effects and may explain why FGAs are not as effective in treating the negative and cognitive effects of schizophrenia. In contrast, SGAs, because they block 5-HT

receptors in addition to DA receptors, give a better clinical profile (control more symptoms) and have fewer adverse effects.

ADVERSE DRUG EFFECTS

Although the incidence and severity of adverse effects may be more tolerable with SGAs than with the older drugs, they are not without adverse effects. In fact, SGAs have some adverse effects not seen with the earlier drugs.

Antipsychotics are notoriously promiscuous drugs. Several, including chlorpromazine (Thorazine), thioridazine (Mellaril), and clozapine (Clozaril), not only block D$_2$ dopamine receptors, but are also antagonists to varying degrees at the D$_1$, D$_2$, and D$_4$ subtypes; 5-HT$_1$ and 5-HT$_2$ receptors; histamine receptors; α_1 and α_2 adrenergic receptors; and M$_1$ and M$_2$ muscarinic cholinergic receptors. This nonspecificity helps explain the breadth of adverse effects associated with antipsychotic drug use. Of all the drugs used to treat schizophrenia, ziprasidone (Geodon) is least likely to produce antimuscarinic symptoms (e.g., dry mouth, blurred vision, constipation, and racing heartbeat). Aripiprazole (Abilify) has the least effect on alpha-1 adrenergic receptors in blood vessels, which can potentially drop blood pressure and make standing up without fainting a challenge (orthostatic hypotension). Prolactinemia is seen with all FGAs and with high doses of risperidone (Risperdal).

One adverse effect that is particularly troubling with the SGAs is weight gain, an effect most frequently seen with clozapine and olanzapine ($\geq$ 7% weight gain in over 40% of patients treated with these two drugs) and least frequently with ziprasidone (Geodon) and aripiprazole (Abilify). Weight gain during treatment is one of the most common reasons for poor patient compliance with SGAs. Moreover, there is also an increase in the incidence of type 2 diabetes mellitus in patients taking SGAs (Baldessarini & Tarazi, 2006). A 10-year study of patients taking clozapine predicted a 43% increase in new-onset type 2 diabetes (Henderson et al., 2005). New-onset diabetes has also been seen to a lesser degree in patients taking risperidone, olanzapine, quetiapine, and ziprasidone. Not enough information is available regarding aripiprazole to know if this drug will have the same effect. To minimize this problem, the Expert Consensus Guidelines (Kane, Leucht, Carpenter, Docherty, & Expert Consensus Panel for Optimizing Pharmacologic Treatment of Psychotic Disorders, 2003) recommends a trial with an antipsychotic with less weight-gain liability when a patient shows clinically significant obesity. The American Diabetes Association recommends a change in antipsychotic drug if the patient gains more than 5% of baseline weight while on the drug (American Diabetes Association, American Psychiatric Association, American Association of Clinical Endocrinology, & North American Association for the Study of Obesity, 2004). It is not clear whether the mechanism for the diabetes development is directly related to the weight gain or vice versa. One study, however, reported that a single dose of a potent 5-HT$_2$-receptor antagonist could alter glucose tolerance and insulin secretion, suggesting that these may be independent effects of the SGAs on body weight (Gilles et al., 2005). Also, SGAs have been shown to increase blood concentrations of lipids and cholesterol and are associated with the onset of myocarditis and cardiomyopathies (Baldessarini & Tarazi, 2006).

Movement disorders are another side effect that can be produced by antipsychotic drugs, particularly the FGAs. The overall incidence of secondary Parkinson's disease or pseudoparkinsonism (extrapyramidal side effects, due to relative imbalance of ACh and DA in the striatum) is fairly common with FGAs, particularly with haloperidol. Of the SGAs, only ziprasidone had a higher incidence of pseudoparkinsonism when compared to a placebo (Gao et al., 2008). Pseudoparkinsonism—if and when it occurs—occurs within days after the patient is put on the drug or soon after the dose is elevated.

Another movement disorder associated with long-term use of antipsychotics is tardive dyskinesia (TD). Rather than appearing early in treatment, TD only occurs after the drug has been used for months to years. In contrast to the extrapyramidal symptoms described above, which dissipate when the drug is discontinued or the dose is lowered, TD may be irreversible or may take years to vanish. The sooner TD is recognized and the sooner the drug is discontinued, the more likely it is to resolve (although not always). With FGAs, the incidence of TD is 5% per year (following the first episode of schizophrenia) (Correll, Leucht, & Kane, 2004). In the elderly, the incidence of TD may be as high as 53% (with 3-year FGA drug treatment.) With SGAs, the incidence is less than 1% per year in nonelderly patients and just a little over 5% with elderly patients. Those numbers, however, overestimate the incidence as almost all patients in these studies had been on FGAs at one time in their lives. The incidence of TD with clozapine is zero. There has never been a report of TD with clozapine. Clozapine is the antipsychotic drug of choice in patients with moderate to severe dyskinesia.

It has also been suggested that the incidence of TD can be minimized in schizophrenic patients by aggressively treating pseudoparkinsonism when it appears. Since this syndrome is due to an imbalance between ACh and DA in the striatum, the clinician has two alternatives: (1) switch to SGAs, which have much less influence in the striatum than FGAs, or (2) add a muscarinic receptor antagonist such as trihexyphenidyl (Artane) to the FGA treatment regimen, to counteract the relative excess of ACh.

If clozapine (Clozaril) is clearly and decisively more effective than FGAs and other SGAs in treatment-resistant schizophrenia, decreases suicide more than other antipsychotics, and does not produce extrapyramidal symptoms or tardive dyskinesia, then why is it not always the drug of first choice for treating schizophrenia? It turns out that clozapine has a rare but nasty side effect, agranulocytosis, a life-threatening condition in which the patient produces an insufficient number of white blood cells (neutrophils or granulocytes) to fight infections. The incidence of agranulocytosis in patients treated with clozapine for 18 months is just 0.9%. While the incidence is rare, the question is, does the benefit outweigh the risk or vice versa? All the SGAs were developed to find a drug as effective as clozapine without this life-threatening side effect. To date, none meet this objective.

DRUG INTERACTIONS

If a patient is put on an antipsychotic, it is essential to take a thorough drug history and look up (online, PDA, or in a book) any potential drug interactions that might alter the dosing regimen or even the drug chosen. Many of the FGAs and SGAs (Table 4-3) are metabolized by cytochrome P450 (CYP) enzymes in the liver, and often by multiple isozymes (CYP 1A2, 2D6 and 3A4, for example). Since these hepatic enzymes metabolize so many other psychotropic and nonpsychotropic drugs, interactions among these drugs are common.

PHARMACOKINETICS

Essentially all of the antipsychotics have long half-lives and can be taken once daily. Ordinarily, once-daily dosing leads to high compliance. However, (out-)patients with schizophrenia are not ordinary patients. They often live alone and lack a support system to assure drug compliance. Although many patients are diligent, others simply cannot or will not take their drugs as prescribed. For these patients depot (slow release) preparations may be necessary. Slow release,

TABLE 4-3 Cytochrome P450 Metabolism

DRUG	MAJOR CYP ISOZYME(S)
First Generation Antipsychotics	
Chlorpromazine	1A2, 2D6
Haloperidol	1A2, 2D6, 3A4
Second Generation Antipsychotics	
Aripiprazole	3A, 2D6
Clozapine	1A2, 3A, 2C19
Olanzapine	1A2, 3A4
Quetiapine	3A4, 2D6
Risperidone	2D6, 3A4
Ziprasidone	3A4

long-acting, intramuscular injections are available for haloperidol (Haldol—monthly), fluphenazine (Prolixin—weekly), and risperidone (Consta—biweekly). The transition of patients from one dosage form to another can be complex and time consuming but is essential to keep these patients functional in an outpatient setting.

PUTTING IT TOGETHER: PART II

Antipsychotic drugs are effective and have been used since the 1950s to free patients from dysfunctional lives filled with anguish. Before the use of antipsychotics these patients were often locked away in human warehouses to either recover or die. Many studies have shown that the one-year relapse rate of schizophrenics is 60% to 80% without drug treatment. With antipsychotics, this rate is between 18% and 32%. With second-generation antipsychotics, the relapse rate is as low as 15% (Crismon, Argo, & Buckley, 2008).

Think about a patient who comes to a mental health practitioner in 2010 with clear signs of schizophrenia, including paranoid delusions, auditory hallucinations, flat affect, avolition, impaired memory, and impaired "executive" function. What is the treatment plan and what drugs should be used to help the schizophrenic patient?

Based on the scientific and clinical evidence, in all likelihood the patient should be started on a single SGA, such as aripiprazole, olanzapine, quetiapine, risperidone, or ziprasidone. If that does not work, and a second SGA is not effective, the next step might be to try clozapine or a FGA. Combinations of a SGA plus a FGA may be needed. In any case, the clinician and the patient have a wide range of drug choices. Given these options are there outside factors that can affect this decision? For example, does—or should—the choice of drug depend on the patient's health insurance coverage? How might the choice be affected if the patient had a prior history of dyskinesia with FGAs? What if the patient is obese and/or diabetic? What if the patient is unlikely to be compliant?

With such a variety of drug choices and other factors to consider, it may be difficult to make a decision. But, in contrast to the state of affairs a half century ago, clinicians' options today have gone from talking, physical restraint, or warehousing, to a relatively wide range of pharmacologic agents that can help patients attain a far greater degree of normalcy than at any time in history. It's a choice worth making.

GENES, BDNF, AND SCHIZOPHRENIA

Because schizophrenia is primarily a disorder in thinking rather than one of mood or memory, if BDNF is involved, the expectation is to find alterations in levels in the cerebral cortex rather than, or in addition to, changes in the limbic system. This, in fact, turns out to be the case. Not only are (prefrontal) cortical levels of BDNF reduced in patients with schizophrenia (Weickert, Hyde, Lipska, Herman, Weinberger, & Kleinman, 2003), but there is evidence that BDNF levels are affected by treatment with antipsychotic drugs (Fumagalli et al., 2003a). Hippocampal levels of BDNF are affected as well in schizophrenic patients (Durany & Thome, 2004). This might

be anticipated given that patients with schizophrenia have difficulty learning from their experiences and often repeat the same detrimental social conduct and judgmental decisions.

In their salient 2003 study, Weickert et al. (Weickert, Hyde, Lipska, Herman, Weinberger, & Kleinman, 2003) reported a 40% BDNF reduction in the dorsolateral prefrontal cortex in autopsies of patients with schizophrenia, when compared to normal cohorts. While this, perhaps, is the clearest evidence of such a relationship, it is merely a correlation, not cause-and-effect. The authors, in fact, raise at least three possible explanations for their findings. First, changes in BDNF may be an epiphenomenon. That is, rather than causing schizophrenia, changes in BDNF might be a consequence of chronic mental illness or the result of treatment. Second, changes in BDNF might be due to inheriting an altered gene for this protein. Third, BDNF levels may fail to rise during some stage of development due to a complex interaction between genetic and environmental factors. Another possibility, not discussed by the Weickert study, is that schizophrenic patients might manufacture an abnormal form of BDNF due to a genetic abnormality. As such, the tissue concentration of BDNF might appear normal, but it might not function properly (see the earlier discussion of Val66Met BDNF polymorphism in Chapter 2). In other words, the Weikert study might actually be underestimating the changes in BDNF function if it only measured the levels of BDNF.

So, which is the correct answer as to why schizophrenic patients have a 40% reduction in BDNF is the dorsolateral prefrontal cortex. Is it choice one, two, three, or four? The answer is that it might be all-of-the-above or none-of-the-above, because no one knows for sure. There is scientific evidence to support all of these options. Remember, brain (hippocampus, specifically) BDNF levels are altered in other mental illnesses in addition to schizophrenia, including major depression, bipolar mood disorder, and Alzheimer's disease. So, changes in BDNF may be an epiphenomenon. Also, several studies suggest that both first- and second-generation antipsychotics can alter BNDF levels, sometimes in an opposing manner (Dawson, Hamid, Egan, & Meredith, 2001; Fumagalli et al., 2003b). The study by Weickert (Weickert et al., 2003) did not distinguish between untreated and treated subjects and, if treated, which type of drug the patient was taking was not noted.

There is much evidence for a genetic component to schizophrenia. For example, while the incidence of schizophrenia in the general population is between 0.6% and 0.9%, the incidence of the illness rises to 10% if a first-degree relative has had it. If both parents have schizophrenia, the incidence increases to 40%; in identical twin studies, if one child has it the likelihood of the disorder appearing in the second is 48% (Crismon et al., 2008). Moreover, based on adoption studies, the risk of schizophrenia lies with the biologic parents, not the adoptive ones. However, despite all this evidence, the genetic component of schizophrenia accounts for only about half the risk and multiple gene loci may be involved (Lewis et al., 2003). Although there is no compelling evidence from family studies of a specific anomaly in the chromosomal region in which the BDNF gene is contained (Egan & Goldberg, 2003), several studies suggest a direct relationship between this gene and the onset of schizophrenia, parietal cortex volume, and incidence of adverse effects in response to antipsychotic drugs.

The third explanation, that BDNF levels fail to rise during some stage of development due to a complex interaction between genetic and environmental factors, is the easiest to accept but the toughest to prove. However, there is a great deal of evidence to support this, especially given the vital role of BDNF in neuronal development. Still—and quite significantly—not all studies have shown a relationship between BDNF and schizophrenia (or other mental illnesses, in fact). It appears that the ethnic makeup of the test population may determine the outcome of the studies (Naoe et al., 2007). Studies done with Caucasian (French, Irish, Scottish) populations have led to different conclusions than those done in Asian (e.g., Chinese, Japanese, Korean) populations. These may be due to differences in detecting a change in a genetic marker or protein, and the specific location of the change, if one is observed. Also, rather than a change in BDNF levels, the difference may show up as an altered BDNF function (effective or not effective; appearance of an EPS adverse effect or not). Perhaps with 50% of the schizophrenic patients (the percent which can be accounted for by genomics), the susceptibility has been laid down before birth. For this group, the genotypic sensitivity only becomes evident (phenotypic) when an (unknown) environmental insult later in life—usually prior to adulthood—unmasks the underlying genomic difference. These insults may range from in utero trauma of some sort to illnesses early in life. Different genes and different environments make finding the precise cause of schizophrenia very difficult. Several dozens, if not hundreds, of genetic polymorphisms have been studied for their relationship to schizophrenia and other mental illnesses, but no individual loci has led to an "aha!" moment (Arranz & de Leon, 2007).

ANTIPSYCHOTICS AND BDNF

Many antipsychotic drugs are metabolized by one or more isozymes of Cytochrome P450 (CYP), the primary oxidative hepatic metabolic pathway for many drugs. Four CYP isozymes (CYP 1A2, 2D6, 2C19, and 3A4) are responsible for metabolizing most antipsychotic drugs (Table 4-3 and Table 4-4). Each of these hepatic enzymes is know to have more than one polymorphism. It has been estimated that there are at least 90 mutations of the gene coding for the CYP 2D6 isozyme, most of which are nonfunctional (Kirchheiner et al., 2004). However, in their review of the literature, Kirchheiner divided patients into four groups based on CYP 2D6 activity (poor, intermediate, extensive, and ultra-rapid metabolizers), and then looked at the clinically effective dose of antipsychotic drug for the patient. For risperidone, the difference in dose between poor and ultra-rapid metabolizers was only 15% (i.e., same dose for all patients), but with olanzapine the clinically effective dose in ultra-rapid metabolizers was as much as three times that seen in the poor metabolizers. This may account for differences in clinical efficacy as well as the incidence of adverse effects among patients, since some patients need very high doses.

Lastly, given that an abnormal form of BDNF, rather than a deficiency in BDNF, is found in some patients with mood disorders, the absence of an association in amount of BDNF and schizophrenia should not automatically imply a lack of a relationship; it just may be harder to uncover. In fact, studies have shown that people with the Val66Val allele of BDNF (the so-called "standard" form) may have a higher incidence of schizophrenia than those with the Val66Met polymorphism (Post, 2007).

So, how does BDNF relate to the hypothetical neurotransmitter (i.e., dopamine) basis of schizophrenia? There are several ways in which these two critical brain chemicals might interact. First, BDNF is a known neurotrophic factor for midbrain dopamine (Goggi, Pullar, Carney, & Bradford, 2003). If lowered BDNF is the initial defect, it might seriously diminish DA innervation of the frontal cortex via the mesocortical pathway. In contrast to the mesolimbic DA pathway, within the mesocortical pathway too little—rather than too much—DA may produce or worsen the negative symptoms of schizophrenia. Alternatively, if the primary impairment is in the DA pathway, this could then reduce BDNF levels. In fact, when rats are injected with either levodopa (the immediate precursor of DA) or with DA-receptor agonists (Guillin et al., 2001), BDNF levels rise. The quest for the relationship between BDNF and mental illness is the proverbial question about which comes first—the chicken or the egg.

TABLE 4-4 Cytochrome P450 Polymorphism

ISOZYME	DRUGS	POLYMORPHISM VARIANT EFFECTS REPORTED
1A2	Chlorpromazine, Haloperidol, Clozapine, Olanzapine	Associated with increased AIMS (Abnormal Involuntary Movement Scale) scores and TD (Tardive dyskinesia), May be interactivity with D3 dopamine receptor subtype polymorphism
2D6	Chlorpromazine, Haloperidol, Aripiprazole, Risperidone	Good predictor of haloperidol adverse effects, ↑ adverse drug reactions with risperidone, larger BMI increases in patients taking olanzapine, associated with TD, EPS, AIMS scores and Parkinsonism in multiple ethnic groups
2C19	Clozapine	No effect on antipsychotic metabolism
3A4	Haloperidol, Aripiprazole, Clozapine, Olanzapine, Quetiapine, Ziprasidone	No connections to effectiveness or adverse effects

62 CHAPTER FOUR

REVIEW QUESTIONS

1. First-generation antipsychotics (FGAs) all effectively block the D_2 subtype of the dopamine receptors. Which of the options below indicate a clinical symptom and an adverse consequence of this interaction in schizophrenic patients?
   a. Reduced positive symptoms and pseudoparkinsonism
   b. Delayed onset of action (weeks) and agranulocytosis
   c. Reduced symptoms of depression in bipolar II patients and tardive dyskinesia
   d. All of the above choices are correct.

2. Of the four main dopamine tracts in the brain, which one is presumed to mediate the positive symptoms of schizophrenia and is the primary site of action of the first-generation antipsychotics (FGAs)?
   a. Nigrostriatal
   b. Tuberoinfundibular
   c. Mesocortical
   d. Mesolimbic

3. If clozapine (Clozaril) is the most clinically effective antipsychotic agent and has an incidence of tardive dyskinesia of zero, why is it not the drug of first choice for treating schizophrenic patients?
   a. High cost to produce
   b. Significantly higher incidence of agranulocytosis than any other antipsychotic drug
   c. Incidence of pseudoparkinsonism in five times higher than with other FGAs or SGAs
   d. Severe orthostatic hypotension (fainting upon standing)

4. What is a common adverse effect of second-generation antipsychotic drug?
   a. Weight gain
   b. Altered glucose tolerance and insulin secretion
   c. Elevated blood cholesterol
   d. All of the above are correct.

5. Albert Hofmann, who discovered LSD, thought that this drug could be used to gain insight into schizophrenia. In what way(s) does the hallucinogenic state induced by LSD differ from the hallucinations of schizophrenic individuals?
   a. LSD hallucinations are due to dopamine and in schizophrenia they are due to 5-HT.
   b. LSD hallucinations are visual in nature whereas in schizophrenia they are generally auditory (hearing voices) in nature.
   c. With LSD hallucinations, people are unaware that they are hallucinating, whereas with schizophrenia patients understand that they are hallucinating
   d. LSD hallucinations are treated with benzodiazepines, whereas treatment of schizophrenic hallucinations is with FGAs or SGAs.

6. Which of the following is not an anatomical pathway utilizing dopamine as a neurotransmitter?
   a. Mesolimbic
   b. Mesocortical
   c. Nigrostriatal
   d. Thalamolimbic

7. Which antipsychotic drug is most likely (0.9% after 18 months) to produce agranulocytosis?
   a. Haloperidol (Haldol)
   b. Fluphenazine (Prolixin)
   c. Clozapine (Clozaril)
   d. Aripiprazole (Abilify)

8. Betty Rubble is an 85-year-old patient who was brought into the emergency room from a nursing home. She is having difficulty following conversations and is paranoid and delusional. Betty has a history of schizophrenia, but she has not required medication for almost 30 years. For the past year or two, however, she has had a resting tremor and may have other symptoms and signs of Parkinson's disease. Which drug listed below might be the drug of first choice for relieving Betty's psychosis?
   a. Haloperidol (Haldol)
   b. Thioridazine (Mellaril)
   c. Escitalopram (Lexapro)
   d. Risperidone (Risperdal)

9. In what two ways do second-generation antipsychotics (SGAs) differ from first-generation antipsychotics (FGAs)?
   a. SGAs are more likely to produce extrapyramidal side effects than are FGAs and they stimulate alpha-1 adrenergic receptors.
   b. SGAs are more likely to produce tardive dyskinesia (TD) than are FGAs and they block $GABA_B$ receptors.
   c. SGAs are less likely to produce extrapyramidal side effects than are FGAs and they block 5-HT receptors.
   d. SGAs are less likely to produce pseudoparkinsonism than are FGAs and they stimulate DA receptors.

10. Janet Renoir is a 35-year-old, nonpregnant patient who is responding well to treatment with haloperidol (Haldol). Recently, however, she has been complaining of breast tenderness, spontaneous lactation, and menstrual irregularities. Blockade of which DA pathway in the brain is most likely responsible for this effect?
    a. Nigrostriatal
    b. Mesocortical
    c. Mesolimbic
    d. Tuberoinfundibular

REFERENCES

American Diabetes Association, American Psychiatric Association, American Association of Clinical Endocrinology, & North American Association for the Study of Obesity. (2004). Consensus development conference on antipsychotic drugs and obesity and diabetes. *Diabetes Care, 27*(2), 596–601.

Arranz, M. J., & de Leon, J. (2007). Pharmacogenetics and pharmacogenomics of schizophrenia: A review of last decade of research. *Molecular Psychiatry, 12*(8), 707–747.

Baldessarini, R. J., & Tarazi, F. I. (2006). Pharmacotherapy of psychosis and mania. In L. L. Brunton, J. S. Lazo, & K. L. Parker (Eds.), *Goodman & Gilman's the pharmacological basis of therapeutics* (11th ed.). New York: McGraw-Hill.

Bleuler, E. (1908). Die prognose der dementia praecox (schizophreniegruppe). *Allg. Z. Psychiatr., 65*, 436–437.

Bleuler, E. (1911). *Dementia praecox oder gruppe der schizophrenien deuticke.* Leipzig: Franz Deuticke.

Correll, C. U., Leucht, S., & Kane, J. M. (2004). Lower risk for tardive dyskinesia associated with second-generation antipsychotics: A systematic review of 1-year studies.[see comment]. *American Journal of Psychiatry, 161*(3), 414–425.

Crismon, M. L., Argo, T. R., & Buckley, P. F. (2008). Schizophrenia. In J. T. DiPiro, R. L. Talbert, G. C. Yee, G. R. Matzke, & B. G. Wells (Eds.), *Pharmacotherapy: A pathophysiologic approach* (7th ed.). New York: McGraw-Hill.

Dawson, N. M., Hamid, E. H., Egan, M. F., & Meredith, G. E. (2001). Changes in the pattern of brain-derived neurotrophic factor immunoreactivity in the rat brain after acute and subchronic haloperidol treatment. *Synapse, 39*(1), 70–81.

Durany, N., & Thome, J. (2004). Neurotrophic factors and the pathophysiology of schizophrenic psychoses. *European Psychiatry: The Journal of the Association of European Psychiatrists, 19*(6), 326–337.

Egan, M. F., & Goldberg, T. E. (2003). Intermediate cognitive phenotypes associated with schizophrenia. *Methods in Molecular Medicine, 77*, 163–197.

Fumagalli, F., Bedogni, F., Maragnoli, M. E., Gennarelli, M., Perez, J., Racagni, G., et al. (2003a). Dopaminergic D2 receptor activation modulates FGF-2 gene expression in rat prefrontal cortex and hippocampus. *Journal of Neuroscience Research, 74*(1), 74–80.

Fumagalli, F., Molteni, R., Roceri, M., Bedogni, F., Santero, R., Fossati, C., et al. (2003b). Effect of antipsychotic drugs on brain-derived neurotrophic factor expression under reduced N-methyl-D-aspartate receptor activity. *Journal of Neuroscience Research, 72*(5), 622–628.

Gao, K., Kemp, D. E., Ganocy, S. J., Gajwani, P., Xia, G., & Calabrese, J. R. (2008). Antipsychotic-induced extrapyramidal side effects in bipolar disorder and schizophrenia: A systematic review. *Journal of Clinical Psychopharmacology, 28*(2), 203–209.

Gilles, M., Wilke, A., Kopf, D., Nonell, A., Lehnert, H., & Deuschle, M. (2005). Antagonism of the serotonin (5-HT)-2 receptor and insulin sensitivity: Implications for atypical antipsychotics. *Psychosomatic Medicine, 67*(5), 748–751.

Goggi, J., Pullar, I. A., Carney, S. L., & Bradford, H. F. (2003). Signalling pathways involved in the short-term potentiation of dopamine release by BDNF. *Brain Research, 968*(1), 156–161.

Guillin, O., Diaz, J., Carroll, P., Griffon, N., Schwartz, J. C., & Sokoloff, P. (2001). BDNF controls dopamine D3 receptor expression and triggers behavioural sensitization. *Nature, 411*(6833), 86–89.

Henderson, D. C., Nguyen, D. D., Copeland, P. M., Hayden, D. L., Borba, C. P., Louie, P. M., et al. (2005). Clozapine, diabetes mellitus, hyperlipidemia, and cardiovascular risks and mortality: Results of a 10-year naturalistic study. *Journal of Clinical Psychiatry, 66*(9), 1116–1121.

Hofmann, A. (1980). *LSD—my problem child.* New York: McGraw-Hill.

Howes, O. D., & Kapur, S. (2009). The dopamine hypothesis of schizophrenia: Version III—The final common pathway. *Schizophr Bull, 35*(3), 549–562.

Kane, J. M., Leucht, S., Carpenter, D., Docherty, J. P., & Expert Consensus Panel for Optimizing Pharmacologic Treatment of Psychotic Disorders. (2003). The expert consensus guideline series. Optimizing pharmacologic treatment of psychotic disorders. Introduction: Methods, commentary, and summary. *Journal of Clinical Psychiatry, 64*(Suppl 12), 5–19.

Kinon, B. J., & Lieberman, J. A. (1996). Mechanisms of action of atypical antipsychotic drugs: A critical analysis. *Psychopharmacology, 124*(1–2), 2–34.

Kirchheiner, J., Nickchen, K., Bauer, M., Wong, M. L., Licinio, J., Roots, I., et al. (2004). Pharmacogenetics of antidepressants and antipsychotics: The contribution of allelic variations to the phenotype of drug response. *Molecular Psychiatry, 9*(5), 442–473.

Kraepelin, E. (1893). *Ein kurzes lehrbuch der psychiatrie. 4 aufl barth,* Lepzig: Barth.

Lewis, C. M., Levinson, D. F., Wise, L. H., DeLisi, L. E., Straub, R. E., Hovatta, I., et al. (2003). Genome scan meta-analysis of schizophrenia and bipolar disorder, part II: Schizophrenia. *American Journal of Human Genetics, 73*(1), 34–48.

Lieberman, J. A., Golden, R., Stroup, S., & McEvoy, J. (2000). Drugs of the psychopharmacological revolution in clinical psychiatry. [see comment]. *Psychiatric Services, 51*(10), 1254–1258.

Lopez-Munoz, F., Alamo, C., Cuenca, E., Shen, W. W., Clervoy, P., & Rubio, G. (2005). History of the discovery and clinical introduction of chlorpromazine. *Annals of Clinical Psychiatry, 17*(3), 113–135.

Morel, B. A. (1852–1853). *Etude cliniques. vol. tom I and II.* Paris: JP Bailliere.

Naoe, Y., Shinkai, T., Hori, H., Fukunaka, Y., Utsunomiya, K., Sakata, S., et al. (2007). No association between the brain-derived neurotrophic factor (BDNF) Val66Met polymorphism and schizophrenia in Asian populations: Evidence from a case-control study and meta-analysis. *Neuroscience Letters, 415*(2), 108–112.

Nestler, E. J., Hyman, S. E., & Malenka, R. C. (2008). *Molecular neuropharmacology: A foundation for clinical neuroscience* (2nd ed.). New York: McGraw-Hill.

Post, R. M. (2007). Role of BDNF in bipolar and unipolar disorder: Clinical and theoretical implications. *Journal of Psychiatric Research, 41*(12), 979–990.

Stahl, S. M. (2008). *Stahl's essential psychopharmacology: Neuroscientific basis and practical applications* (3rd ed.). New York: Cambridge University Press.

Tardive dyskinesia—definition, description, causes and symptoms, demographics, treatments, prognosis. Retrieved 5/10/2009, 2009, from http://www.minddisorders.com/Py-Z/Tardive-dyskinesia. html

Weickert, C. S., Hyde, T. M., Lipska, B. K., Herman, M. M., Weinberger, D. R., & Kleinman, J. E. (2003). Reduced brain-derived neurotrophic factor in prefrontal cortex of patients with schizophrenia. *Molecular Psychiatry, 8*(6), 592–610.

Whitaker, R. (2003). *Mad in America: Bad science, bad medicine, and the enduring mistreatment of the mentally ill.* Cambridge, MA: Da Capo Press.

CHAPTER 5
Cognitive Enhancers

If a kid asks where rain comes from, I think a cute thing to tell him is "God is crying."
And if he asks why God is crying, another cute thing to tell him is "probably because of
something you did."

JACK HANDY

GETTING PERSONAL

From an early age we knew our son, Willie, was different. Even as a baby, he never slept well. Most nights he was awake at least a couple of times during the night and he rarely took more than one nap per day. As a toddler and to this day he's always been extremely spirited and active. In fact, as an example, he is now 9 years old and he has never been able to sit with us through an entire meal.

Transitioning from one activity to another has always been and is still difficult. It usually results in a major temper tantrum and a lot of uncontrollable anger. Willie gets very physical, not only with our home (throwing and kicking things, slamming doors) but with us, as well (kicking, hitting, screaming, name calling). Traditional discipline methods such as time-outs and consequences have not been effective.

When Willie was 4 years old we had him evaluated. Eventually he was diagnosed with moderate to severe ADHD (Attention Deficit Hyperactivity Disorder). In kindergarten his teacher talked to us about having to redirect him often.

She regularly used the saying "Hocus Pocus, it's time to focus"—to get him back on track. Based on her observations, she recommended we look into an IEP plan (Individual Education Plan). We met with the principal, our son's kindergarten teacher, and the special education instructor and learned that he was indeed eligible for an IEP plan. This news was very bittersweet. It really hit home—the sad and true reality was that we had a child that needed special attention, but on the other hand, here was a program that would help him along the way. Our son is very bright and didn't need help intellectually or academically. He needed help with staying on task, staying focused, and with some social issues (he would often speak out of turn, disrupting the activity of the moment and he didn't have a clue what personal space was). The IEP plan started in first grade.

In addition to the IEP plan, we worked with Willie's psychologist and psychiatrist. Midway through the school year our psychiatrist recommended we try medication. We were extremely skeptical and uncomfortable with the idea of using drugs. We did a lot of research and talked with many parents and professionals about the pros and cons before determining whether or not it was the right thing to do. Willie started on Ritalin, but it made him so sad and withdrawn. We ended up changing the medication to Adderall XR, with better results.

Through the rest of first grade, with the help of the IEP program, regular meetings with his psychologist for behavioral issues, and the Adderall, we saw much improvement. The report cards and comments we received from his teacher and the special education staff were very positive. During the school day he was staying on track and his attention span was much better. Willie didn't need to be redirected as often and he was making friends. In fact we would often hear that he would step in, as a peacemaker or in defense of another classmate when there was a conflict. We continued the same course of treatment through second grade with great results. In fact, at the end of the school year it was decided that he no longer needed the IEP program. This was great news.

Of course, there are some negative side affects with using drugs. One of the things that we notice while Willie is on Adderall is that his personality is "zapped." He becomes very withdrawn and any enthusiasm or excitement disappears. I describe it as "flat-lined." Another negative is that the medication causes a lack of appetite. So, he eats very little during the day, which concerns us from a nutritional standpoint. We are also worried about the long-term effects of stimulant drugs on brain development and other issues that might arise in the future.

Willie is now nearing the end of third grade. At one point earlier in the school year it was recommended that we try a new medication called Vyvanse. There was a possibility that it wouldn't make him seem so withdrawn, but because the effects lasted past dinner and caused a lack of appetite, we stopped using it. After this we thought we'd try a test and intentionally decided not to put him back on Adderall, just to see if there was a difference in school. We didn't tell his teacher. One day, within the first week without medication, she pulled us aside and said she had to speak with him often about staying on track and not being disruptive and that she had to redirect him a lot. It was clear that the medication helped him. Willie and his teacher like each other so much (I call it a love affair). His principal recently said to us, "We wish our school had more Willies!" He's having a great year. He has a lot of friends and enjoys team sports and is playing basketball and baseball.

I used to think ADHD was just an excuse for poor parenting, but that is no longer the case. Raising a child with ADHD has a lot of challenges and is really difficult. But there is definitely hope and many resources are available to help us.

We still meet with our psychologist and psychiatrist on a monthly basis. We hope that as Willie matures, maybe one day he won't need the medication. But at this point, there is no question that the medication is helping. We will continue the combined treatment schedule, as we believe there has been a great improvement in our son's life and in our lives too.

Anonymous

NO MAGIC PILL

Combine having a bad memory and being unable to concentrate and then amplify these issues many times over. The resulting clinical situations will mirror the functionally disabling illnesses of Alzheimer's disease (named for Alois Alzheimer) and attention deficit hyperactivity disorder (ADHD). Doesn't every sentient soul with a child or parent suffering from these disorders wish there were a pill to cure them? While there is no magic pill, there are some drugs available that can help modify some of the symptoms of ADHD and Alzheimer's disease.

This chapter focuses on the specific pharmacologic agents to enhance attention for ADHD patients (stimulants) and memory for Alzheimer's disease (AD) patients (cholinesterase inhibitors).

ATTENTION DEFICIT HYPERACTIVITY DISORDER (ADHD)

ADHD affects 5% to 10% of school-age children. The symptoms persist into adolescence in about 60% to 80% of these cases, and for 30% to 40% it continues into adulthood

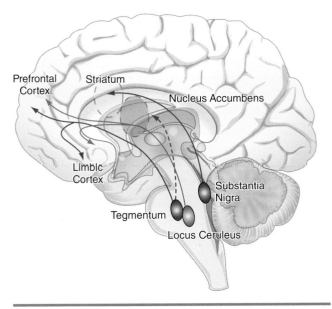

FIGURE 5-1 Major NE pathways (orange) running from the locus ceruleus to the prefrontal and limbic cortex. Major DA pathways (blue, covered in detail in Chapter 4). The DA pathways are believed to be involved with attention (solid blue lines) and run from the tegmentum to the prefrontal and limbic cortex. Also shown (dashed blue line) is the mesolimbic pathway, running from the ventral tegmentum to the nucleus accumbens.

(Mannuzza & Klein, 2000). Inattentiveness, inability to control impulsive behaviors, and hyperactivity denote the classic symptom triad of ADHD. Two neurotransmitters, norepinephrine and dopamine, are believed to play active roles in these dysfunctions. Figure 5-1 shows the neuroanatomical localization of the major NE and DA brain pathways involved in attention (solid lines) and Table 5-1 shows functions and behaviors mediated by these neurotransmitters (Stahl, 2008).

As noted below, changes in NE and DA levels in the prefrontal and limbic cortex mediate the therapeutic effects—and some adverse effects—of ADHD drugs.

Assuming that the prefrontal (NE) and mesocortical (DA) pathways are involved in maintaining and focusing attention, it is easy to imagine how deficient NE and/or DA activity in these two key pathways might lead to many of the primary signs and symptoms of ADHD (e.g., hyperactivity, impulsivity, and inattention) as well as many of the secondary symptoms (e.g., disorganization, inability to plan, difficulty controlling emotions, poor time management). It is also easy to see how raising the levels of DA and NE would reduce the symptoms of ADHD. In fact, this is the mode of action of all drugs used to treat ADHD.

Other than atomoxetine (Straterra), the drugs used to treat ADHD are central nervous system stimulants (psychostimulants) (Merck Research Laboratories, 2006). Drugs such as methylphenidate and amphetamines are effective in 80% to 90% of children with ADHD and are first-line treatments for ADHD (The MTA Cooperative Group, 1999). The stimulant drugs (Table 5-2) include amphetamines in immediate-release (Dexedrine) or sustained-release (Dexedrine Spansules, and Adderall XR) formulations, and methylphenidate in immediate-release (Ritalin) or sustained-release (Concerta and Metadate CD) formulations. The advantage of the sustained-release preparations is that they are sufficiently long acting that they only need be administered in the morning. From a practical standpoint they do not need to be administered during school hours, removing the burden on schools to manage drug administration.

All these drugs have similar neurochemical actions (Westfall & Westfall, 2006) in that they enhance DA and/or NE release and block their reuptake. Methylphenidate and d-amphetamine affect DA neurons primarily and d,l-amphetamine also affects NE release. This makes perfect sense except for one small thing . . . it is completely counterintuitive.

Why do CNS stimulants help ADHD at all? Why should a stimulant improve attention, diminish impulsivity, decrease hyperactivity, and seemingly calm the patient? It seems like the opposite would occur—that a stimulant would worsen ADHD. What is the logical approach to this conundrum?

There are at least two reasons why this might happen. First, areas of the prefrontal and limbic cortex involved with focusing and maintaining attention and prioritizing behaviors

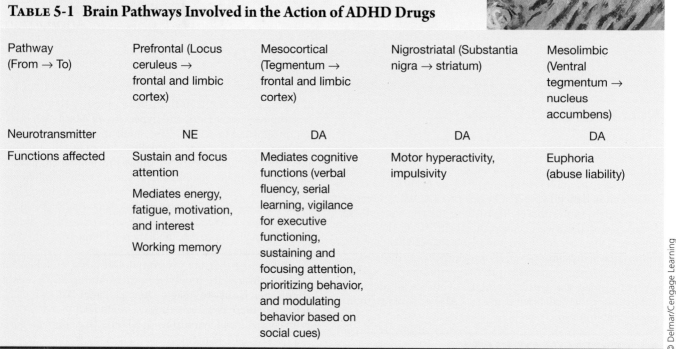

TABLE 5-1 Brain Pathways Involved in the Action of ADHD Drugs

Pathway (From → To)	Prefrontal (Locus ceruleus → frontal and limbic cortex)	Mesocortical (Tegmentum → frontal and limbic cortex)	Nigrostriatal (Substantia nigra → striatum)	Mesolimbic (Ventral tegmentum → nucleus accumbens)
Neurotransmitter	NE	DA	DA	DA
Functions affected	Sustain and focus attention Mediates energy, fatigue, motivation, and interest Working memory	Mediates cognitive functions (verbal fluency, serial learning, vigilance for executive functioning, sustaining and focusing attention, prioritizing behavior, and modulating behavior based on social cues)	Motor hyperactivity, impulsivity	Euphoria (abuse liability)

are activated by psychostimulants at low (therapeutic) doses (Farone & Biederman, 2002). At higher doses, areas of the brain involved in motor activity and arousal are activated. In other words, at the therapeutic doses used for ADHD these drugs improve focus and attentiveness but the drugs do act as stimulants with higher doses.

Second, amphetamine-like stimulants have three dose-related actions on neurotransmission. The lowest doses of these drugs facilitate the amount of NE and DA released by action potentials reaching the axon terminal, increasing the amount of transmitter that can act on postsynaptic receptors. With higher doses, NE and DA reuptake at the neuron is blocked, further elevating NE or DA levels. At very high doses, the intraneuronal enzyme monoamine oxidase (MAO) is inhibited, raising the neurotransmitter levels even higher.

It also may be that patients with ADHD are somehow "wired" differently. Not only do stimulants have a calming action in patients with ADHD but tolerance also develops at a slower pace than in non-ADHD patients. In addition, people who abuse amphetamines (and cocaine) often develop "reverse tolerance" and may become psychotic with chronic use of the drug, even without dose escalation. ADHD patients do not display this action.

TABLE 5-2 CNS Stimulant Pharmacokinetics

MEDICATION	BRAND	FREQUENCY	PEAK EFFECT	DURATION OF ACTION
d-Amphetamine	Dexedrine	2 or 3 times per day	1–3 hours	5 hours
d-Amphetamine	Dexedrine Spansules	Once in AM	1–4 hours	6–9 hours
d,l-Amphetamine	Adderall	2 or 3 times per day	1–3 hours	5 hours
d,l-Amphetamine	Adderall XR	Once in AM	1–4 hours	9 hours
Methylphenydate	Ritalin	3 times per day	1–3 hours	2–4 hours
d-Methylphenydate	Focalin	2 times per day	1–4 hours	2–5 hours
Methylphenydate	Ritalin SR	1 or 2 times a day	3 hours	5 hours
Methylphenydate	Metadate CD	Once in AM	5 hours	8 hours
Methylphenydate	Concerta	Once in AM	8 hours	12 hours

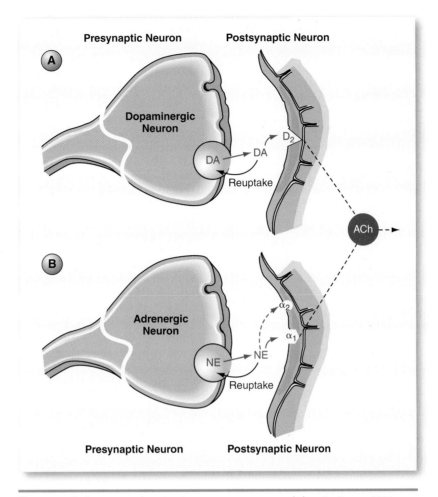

FIGURE 5-2 Release of DA by dopaminergic neurons (A) and release of NE by adrenergic neurons (B) increase the levels of ACh in the prefrontal cortex, improving memory in ADHD patients.

Atomoxetine (Strattera), a highly selective NE reuptake inhibitor, is the only first-line ADHD medication that has no abuse potential and is not a DEA Schedule II controlled substance. It does not directly affect DA levels in the nucleus accumbens, the area of the brain that mediates the euphoric properties (i.e., abuse liability) of psychostimulants. As such, it is the only drug approved by the FDA to treat adult ADHD. Interestingly, for reasons not readily apparent, this selective NE-reuptake inhibitor not only elevates NE levels in the prefrontal cortex, it also elevates DA levels there but not in the nucleus accumbens or the striatum.

A report by Tzavara and coworkers (Tzavara et al., 2006) offers additional insight into the clinical efficacy of atomoxetine. Difficulties in working memory are a common problem in ADHD patients. Although cholinergic (ACh) neurons impacting upon cortical and subcortical regions of the brain are implicated in vigilance, attention, and working memory, the impact of atomoxetine and methylphenidate on ACh neurotransmission in this part of the brain has not been studied adequately. Using highly selective receptor antagonists for NE and DA, Tzavara and colleagues (2006) observed that atomoxetine and methylphenidate increased ACh release in rat brain frontal cortex only when both α_1-NE receptors and D_1-DA receptors were activated by synaptic NE and DA that was

released by atomoxetine or methylphenidate. Moreover, this effect was consistent with the time course of improvement in working memory produced by the drugs. These data suggest yet another neurochemical mechanism to explain the therapeutic benefits of atomoxetine and methylphenidate. That is, the overall improvement in attention and memory seen with both drugs is due to the combined rise in NE, DA, and ACh levels in the prefrontal cortex (Figure 5-2). Although the role of ACh in improving memory in ADHD patients is just beginning to be appreciated, the critical role of this transmitter, particularly its loss in Alzheimer's disease, is well established.

ALZHEIMER'S DISEASE (AD)

Alzheimer's disease (AD) is the consequence of cortical degeneration. Its signature symptom is dementia, a progressive loss of cognitive function. The disease usually comes to light when patients show impaired higher intellectual function with altered mood and behavior. As it progresses, disorientation, memory loss, and aphasia may occur. AD is rare in the young and is the most common form of dementia in the elderly. The prevalence of AD goes from 1% to 40% or more between the ages of 60 and 90.

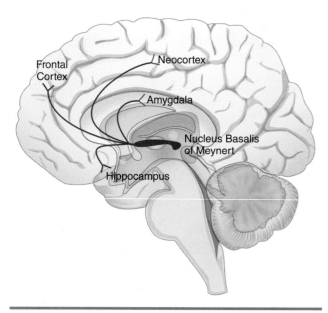

FIGURE 5-3 Four key cholinergic pathways in the brain originating in the nucleus basalis of Meynert and going to the (1) neocortex, (2) amygdala, (3) hippocampus, and (4) frontal cortex.

Many symptoms of Alzheimer's disease (AD), particularly those involving memory, are due to the destruction of cholinergic neurons in several areas of the brain. The nucleus basalis of Meynert (NBM) is the brain center where many cholinergic (ACh) neuron cell bodies originate (Figure 5-3), and it is where the earliest damage to the brain in AD is thought to occur (Whitehouse et al., 1982).

The uniqueness of AD lies in its hallmark pathology. As Alzheimer and Kraepelin discovered early in the last century, when viewed macroscopically the autopsied brain of the AD patient shows cortical atrophy primarily in cholinergic neurons innervating the frontal, temporal, and parietal lobes. There are two key microscopic changes that occur as well.

Neurofibrillary tangles filled with structurally incompetent tau protein begin to form and surround the neuron's microtubules. (Figure 5-4, part B). These tangles interfere with the cell's ability to transport essential chemicals along the microtubules from the cell body, down the axon to the terminals. The congested conveyor eventually results in cell death.

At the same time, on the exterior of NBM neurons, β-amyloid polypeptides are overproduced and accumulate in the synapse. This, too, interferes with normal cholinergic neurotransmission and the first signs of memory loss are observed. Over time, the damage becomes more widespread and additional areas of the brain innervated by the NBM (e.g., hippocampus and amygdala) begin to die off. As the disease continues to progress, diffuse damage to the neocortex occurs.

Memory problems in AD patients coincide with neuronal loss in the NBM (Figure 5-5). Within approximately three years, as cell damage and loss spreads to areas of the brain receiving cholinergic innervation from the NBM (e.g., hippocampus and amygdala, entorhinal cortex), the patient loses functional independence and an early diagnosis

of AD can be made. Three to six years later, the neocortex is heavily involved in the disease process and the patient generally needs to be placed in a nursing home to assure proper care. With few exceptions these patients die over the ensuing three years.

Although no treatment has been shown to "cure" Alzheimer's patients, one class of drugs, the cholinesterase inhibitors, delays the progression of the disease, to varying degrees. This class of drugs delays cognitive deterioration by one year in approximately 20% of treated patients (DeLaGarza, 2003). However, although these drugs seem to be somewhat effective in treating AD patients, they raise ACh levels throughout the brain, not just in areas where the transmitter levels are deficient. As such, these drugs have many adverse effects (e.g., nausea, anorexia, vomiting, and diarrhea) that limit the maximal dose that can be used clinically.

When mitochondrial Acetyl-Coenzyme A combines with intracellular choline, with the help of the enzyme choline acetyltransferase, it forms ACh, which is taken up into vesicles and released following an action potential in the cell (Figure 5-4 part A). Once released, ACh can act on either nicotinic or muscarinic receptor subtypes. The M_1-muscarinic subtype plays a distinct, well-defined role in memory, although other ACh receptors may play some role as well. Importantly, ACh is rapidly (in several millionths of a second) broken down in the synapse by the enzyme acetylcholinesterase (AChE). A second enzyme, butyrylcholinesterase (BuChE), found mostly outside the CNS and within glial cells inside the CNS, can metabolize any ACh that diffuses away from the synapse. BuChE does not normally play a role in neurotransmission, since it is not located in the synapse.

CHOLINESTERASE (AChE) INHIBITORS

All drugs used to treat mild to moderate AD elevate ACh levels by inhibiting acetylcholinesterase (AChE), acetylcholine's primary degradative enzyme. As a class, they are referred to as cholinesterase inhibitors. They include donepezil (Aricept), galantamine (Razadyne, formerly known as Reminyl), and rivastigmine (Exelon). The most common adverse effects of these drugs are transient gastrointestinal issues.

Because tacrine (Cognex) has a short half-life (i.e., it needs to be given multiple times per day), has many drug interactions (especially NSAIDs), and may cause liver damage, it is now considered second-line therapy for AD. Donepezil (Aricept) has the advantage of a longer half-life (once daily administration vs. four times per day for tacrine).

Rivastagmine (Exelon) inhibits both AChE and BuChE and it only needs to be administered twice daily, which results in good compliance. Unlike the other cholinesterase inhibitors, however, it may cause gastrointestinal problems and muscle weakness.

Galantamine (Razadyne) inhibits AChE and stimulates nicotinic cholinergic neurons to release more stored ACh. This drug should be taken cautiously in patients taking the antidepressants paroxetine, amitriptyline, fluoxetine, and fluvoxamine as well as drugs with anticholinergic side effects, as these drugs may interfere with the elimination of galantamine from the body.

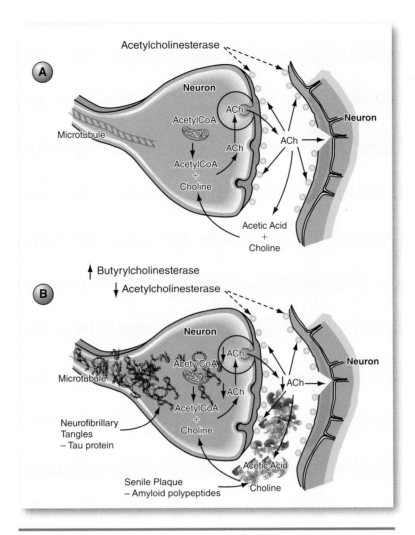

FIGURE 5-4 Panel A shows a normally functioning cholinergic neuron. Precursor chemicals are transported from the cell body along the axon via microtubules to the terminal. Acetylcholine (ACh) is released into the synapse where it can act on receptors, diffuse away, or be metabolized. In panel B neurons damage by AD are shown with neurofibrillatory tangles and amyloid polypeptides.

A drug that may be useful in patients with moderate to severe AD is memantine (Namenda), an antagonist at the NMDA subtype of glutamate (GLU) receptor. In clinical studies this drug has been found to help patients in the later stages of the disease to maintain additional independence. The most common adverse effects of memantine are dizziness, headache, constipation, and confusion.

Other drugs that have been evaluated as potential treatments for AD include Vitamin E, selegiline (Eldepryl), estrogen, NSAIDs, and ginkgo biloba. Despite numerous studies with Vitamin E, there is insufficient evidence to recommend its use for AD. The same is true for selegiline, a monoamine oxidase inhibitor sometimes used in the treatment of Parkinson's disease. While estrogen may have a neuroprotective effect, again, there is no evidence that it improves cognition or function in AD patients. Likewise, anti-inflammatory drugs may be somewhat neuroprotective but do not show benefit for treatment. Ginkgo biloba may have a modest benefit for AD patients but serious side effects (bleeding, seizures, coma) have been reported with commercial pharmaceutical-grade ginkgo biloba preparations (which are unavailable in the US). Moreover, a 2008 randomized, double-blind, placebo controlled clinical trial with over three thousand volunteers (DeKosky et al., 2008) found no beneficial effect of the herb on any tests of memory, thinking, and personality nor did it alter the course of dementia and AD.

One interesting direction of AD research deals with apolipoprotein E (Bu, 2009). Lipoproteins are proteins associated with fat. Apolipoprotein E (ApoE) is a component of very low-density lipoproteins (VLDL) that help remove cholesterol from blood and transport it to the liver for metabolism and low-density lipoproteins (LDL), which helps deposit cholesterol onto vascular walls (very bad for

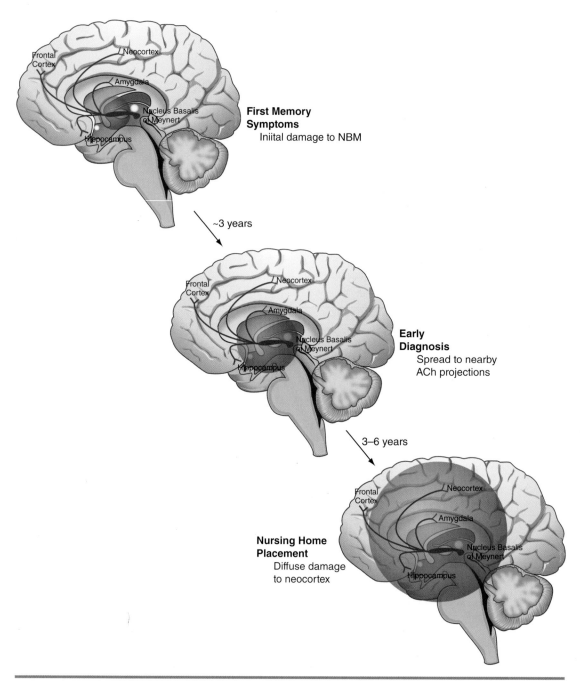

First Memory Symptoms
Iniital damage to NBM

~3 years

Early Diagnosis
Spread to nearby ACh projections

3–6 years

Nursing Home Placement
Diffuse damage to neocortex

FIGURE 5-5 Time course of neuropathologic damage in Alzheimer's disease damage relative to symptom onset and duration of illness. Maroon circles in this image show the progressive course of neuropathic damage in Alzheimer's disease relative to symptom onset and duration of illness.

vascular health). Three genes code-for ApoE (e2 [actually ε2], e3, and e4, with e3 alleles being most common and e4 occurring in about 15% of the population) and everyone has two versions of the ApoE lipoprotein. Therefore, it is possible for an individual to have any one of six possible combinations (ApoE phenotypes E2/2, E2/3, E2/4, E3/3, E3/4 and E4/4).

This information is important because ApoE is also present in the brain, and research done over the last few years suggests that it may play a vital role in both the development of AD and its response to treatment. Specifically, patients with sporadic and late-onset AD were found to have an unusually high frequency of the e4 allele. Poirier (1999) reported that AD patients with one or two copies of the e4 allele had lower levels of choline acetyltransferase (ChAT) and nicotinic ACh binding sites in both the hippocampus and the temporal cortex. Those patients with two copies of ApoE e4 had significantly fewer neurons in their NBM than AD patients with no e4 alleles (e4 negative). In addition, cholinesterase inhibitors were found to be more effective in 44 negative AD patients, whereas other AD drugs were more effective in e-4 carriers.

BDNF AND AD

This chapter is not complete without at least a brief discussion of brain-derived neurotrophic factor (BDNF). As noted in earlier chapters, this neurotrophic factor is involved with memory in the hippocampus and other areas of the brain. As memory defects are a hallmark symptom of AD, BDNF might be a logical target for investigation to develop more effective treatment strategies of AD (Hubka, 2006). Interestingly, the areas of the AD brain with the greatest decreases in BDNF signaling (BDNF content and TrkB receptors) are the hippocampus, frontal, temporal, parietal, and entorhinal cortices; these are the areas of the brain most impaired in AD (Murer, Yan, & Raisman-Vozari, 2001). Furthermore, all drugs effective in treating AD directly affect or up-regulate BDNF signaling pathways. Leyhe (Leyhe, Stransky, Eschweiler, Buchkremer, & Laske, 2008) has suggested that up-regulation of BDNF might be part of a neuroprotective effect of AChE-inhibitors, perhaps by blocking the toxic effects of amyloid beta proteins (Arancibia et al., 2008).

If BDNF and other neurotrophins are neuroprotective and represent a potential treatment target for neurodegenerative disorders, why not administer them directly to patients? One problem, as noted by Shulte-Herbruggen (Schulte-Herbruggen, Braun, Rochlitzer, Jockers-Scherubl, & Hellweg, 2007) is that in humans neurotrophin administration induces severe side effects such as pain and weight loss—and thus the risk outweighs the potential benefits. In the future, studies that administer the drug into the brain locally (rather than systemically) may yield more favorable outcomes.

ACETYLCHOLINE (ACh) IN ADHD AND AD

Both ADHD and AD patients have defects in areas of the brain that result in cognitive dysfunction, including, but not limited to, memory processing. Decades of research have shown that CNS stimulants, drugs that elevate both NE and DA in the prefrontal cortex, improve cognitive function in ADHD patients. Only recently, however, has the role of acetylcholine in this disorder been investigated, and the results look promising. One of the major drawbacks of the psychostimulants is their high abuse liability. Atomoxetine, a highly selective NE reuptake blocker, which indirectly elevates DA in the cortex, but not the nucleus accumbens, may also elevate ACh levels. This drug, while only moderately effective in treating ADHD, has no abuse liability.

Interestingly, drugs that elevate ACh are the hallmarks of treatment of Alzheimer's disease. They have been shown conclusively to delay functional loss in AD patients, by as much as several years, but are ineffective in other patients. Recent pharmacogenetic studies suggest that poor responders to cholinesterase inhibitors may be carriers for a specific lipoprotein (ApoE e4) that is associated with several abnormalities in ACh function in critical areas of the brain. Perhaps there will be new cholesterol medications designed specifically to improve brain function. In any event, the pursuit of new drugs to treat ADHD and AD will continue with the hope of finding even more effective drugs to help patients suffering from these disorders.

REVIEW QUESTIONS

1. ADHD is a childhood illness that dissipates as the patient moves through adolescence into adulthood.
   a. True
   b. False

2. Which pathway, involved in the action of drugs used to treat ADHD, utilizes norepinephrine (NE) rather than dopamine (DA) as the neurotransmitter?
   a. Locus ceruleus → frontal and limbic cortex
   b. Tegmentum → frontal and limbic cortex
   c. Substantia nigra → striatum
   d. Ventral tegmentum → nucleus accumbens

3. Which of the following drugs used to treat ADHD is least likely to be abused and is not a DEA Schedule II controlled substance?
   a. Immediate release d-amphetamine (Dexedrine)
   b. Sustained release d,l-amphetamine (Adderall XR)
   c. Sustained release methylphenidate (Concerta)
   d. Atomoxetine (Straterra)

4. In patients with Alzheimer's disease (AD), when do memory problems first begin to appear?
   a. With neuronal loss in the nucleus basalis of Meynert (NBM)
   b. When neurofibrillatory tangles occur in the substantia nigra
   c. Generally, two years after treatment with an anticholinesterase is initiated
   d. Only when the neocortex becomes involved

5. What limits the maximum dose of drug that can be used to treat AD patients?
   a. Progression of the disease
   b. Insurance coverage
   c. Adverse effects
   d. Maximal drug efficacy reached (i.e., when all receptors are occupied)

6. Which dopamine (DA) pathway, involved in the action of drugs used to treat ADHD, contributes to the abuse liability of most drugs in this class?
   a. Locus ceruleus → frontal and limbic cortex
   b. Tegmentum → frontal and limbic cortex
   c. Substantia nigra → striatum
   d. Ventral tegmentum → nucleus accumbens

7. Which of the following drugs for ADHD is administered only once daily, in the morning?
   a. d-amphetamine (Dexedrine Spansules)
   b. d,l-amphetamine (Adderall XR)
   c. Methylphenidate (Concerta)
   d. All of the above

8. What is the only FDA approved drug to treat adult ADHD?
   a. Atomoxetine (Strattera)
   b. d-amphetamine (Dexedrine Spansules)
   c. d,l-amphetamine (Adderall XR)
   d. Methylphenidate (Concerta)

9. What two pathophysiological changes are characteristic of Alzheimer's disease?
   a. Degeneration of the substantia nigra and elevated levels of P-glycoprotein
   b. Accumulation of beta-amyloid polypeptides and increased hippocampal neurogenesis
   c. Decreased apoptosis and neuroplasticity in the neocortex and the nucleus basalis of Meynert
   d. Neurofibrillary tangles in the cerebral cortex and accumulation of beta-amyloid polypeptides in nucleus basalis of Meynert synapses

10. Which of the following drugs is not used to treat the cognitive and memory problems associated with Alzheimer's disease?
    a. Venlafaxine (Effexor)
    b. Tacrine (Cognex)
    c. Donepezil (Aricept)
    d. Rivastigmine (Exelon)

REFERENCES

Arancibia, S., Silhol, M., Mouliere, F., Meffre, J., Hollinger, I., Maurice, T., et al. (2008). Protective effect of BDNF against beta-amyloid induced neurotoxicity in vitro and in vivo in rats. *Neurobiology of Disease, 31*(3), 316–326.

Bu, G. (2009). Apolipoprotein E and its receptors in Alzheimer's disease: Pathways, pathogenesis and therapy. *Nature Reviews Neuroscience, 10*(5), 333–344.

DeLaGarza, V. W. (2003). Pharmacologic treatment of Alzheimer's disease: An update. *American Family Physician, 68*(7), 1365–1372.

DeKosky S. T., Williamson, J. D., Fitzpatrick, A. L., et al. (2008). Ginkgo biloba for prevention of dementia: A randomized controlled trial. *JAMA, 300*(19), 2253–2262.

Farone, S. V., & Biederman, J. (2002). Pathophysiology of attention-deficit hyperactivity disorder. In K. L. Davis, D. Charney, J. T. Coyle, & C. Nemeroff (Eds.), *Neuropsychopharmacology: The fifth generation of progress. An official publication of the American College of Neuropsychopharmacology* (pp. 577–596). Philadelphia: Lippincott Williams & Wilkins.

Hubka, P. (2006). Neural network plasticity, BDNF and behavioral interventions in Alzheimer's disease. *Bratislavske Lekarske Listy, 107*(9–10), 395–401.

Leyhe, T., Stransky, E., Eschweiler, G. W., Buchkremer, G., & Laske, C. (2008). Increase of BDNF serum concentration during donepezil treatment of patients with early Alzheimer's disease. *European Archives of Psychiatry & Clinical Neuroscience, 258*(2), 124–128.

Mannuzza, S., & Klein, R. G. (2000). Long-term prognosis in attention-deficit/hyperactivity disorder. *Child & Adolescent Psychiatric Clinics of North America, 9*(3), 711–726.

Merck Research Laboratories. (2006). Learning and developmental disorders. In M. H. Beers, R. S. Porter, T. V. Jones, J. L. Kaplan, & M. Berkwits (Eds.), *The Merck manual of diagnosis and therapy*, (18th ed.). New Jersey: Merck Research Laboratories.

Murer, M. G., Yan, Q., & Raisman-Vozari, R. (2001). Brain-derived neurotrophic factor in the control human brain, and in Alzheimer's disease and Parkinson's disease. *Progress in Neurobiology, 63*(1), 71–124.

Poirier, J. (1999). Apolipoprotein E4, cholinergic integrity and the pharmacogenetics of Alzheimer's disease.[see comment]. *Journal of Psychiatry & Neuroscience, 24*(2), 147–153.

Schulte-Herbruggen, O., Braun, A., Rochlitzer, S., Jockers-Scherubl, M. C., & Hellweg, R. (2007). Neurotrophic factors—A tool for therapeutic strategies in neurological, neuropsychiatric and neuroimmunological diseases? *Current Medicinal Chemistry, 14*(22), 2318–2329.

Stahl, S. M. (2008). *Stahl's essential psychopharmacology: Neuroscientific basis and practical applications* (3rd ed.). New York: Cambridge University Press.

The MTA Cooperative Group. (1999). A 14-month randomized clinical trial of treatment strategies for attention-deficit/hyperactivity disorder. the MTA cooperative group. multimodal treatment study of children with ADHD. *Archives of General Psychiatry, 56*(12), 1073–1086.

Tzavara, E. T., Bymaster, F. P., Overshiner, C. D., Davis, R. J., Perry, K. W., Wolff, M., et al. (2006). Procholinergic and memory enhancing properties of the selective norepinephrine uptake inhibitor atomoxetine. *Molecular Psychiatry, 11*(2), 187–195.

Westfall, T. C., & Westfall, D. P. (2006). Adrenergic agonists and antagonists. In L. S. Goodman, A. Gilman, L. L. Brunton, J. S. Lazo, & K. L. Parker (Eds.), *Goodman & Gilman's the pharmacological basis of therapeutics* (11th ed.). New York: McGraw-Hill.

Whitehouse, P. J., Price, D. L., Struble, R. G., Clark, A. W., Coyle, J. T., & Delon, M. R. (1982). Alzheimer's disease and senile dementia: Loss of neurons in the basal forebrain. *Science, 215*(4537), 1237–1239.

CHAPTER 6

Anxiolytic–Sedative–Hypnotic Drug Pharmacotherapy

"Innately, children seem to have little true realistic anxiety. They will run along the brink of water, climb on the window sill, play with sharp objects and with fire, in short, do everything that is bound to damage them and to worry those in charge of them, that is wholly the result of education; for they cannot be allowed to make the instructive experiences themselves."

SIGMUND FREUD

GETTING PERSONAL

While writing this book, I contacted friends, relatives, and professional colleagues to help me gather vignettes from patients with the mental illnesses discussed throughout this book. Overall, this worked quite well but there was one topic where I could get no assistance. The topic was anxiety, particularly generalized anxiety disorder. Everyone who spoke to their friends, colleagues, and patients with this condition came back with the same answer, no dice. The people they had turned to, who they thought could express themselves in writing, would not do so, ironically because of anxiety. Despite my assurances of anonymity these individuals were afraid that they would be exposed or revealed and their lives would be ruined (again).

At one point I was going to write the vignette myself for, as the submission date for the final copy of my manuscript loomed prominently, I began experiencing daily bouts of anxiety and occasional panic attacks. I feared that I would be missing a key element of the book, since I could not get this one vignette done. I would wake up early, and fall asleep late and worried throughout the day about this issue. I could not let it go. I could not stop worrying. I was hung up on this one item and couldn't proceed.

Two things finally helped, a month of alprazolam (Xanax) and recognizing that I could turn this problem into strength by addressing rather than ignoring it. My difficulties in building this vignette in fact exemplified the seriousness of an anxiety disorder. I came to appreciate just how debilitating anxiety disorders can be. I took it for granted that the anxiety vignette would be the easiest one to get, but it turned out to be the most difficult. Studies have shown that people are more willing to admit addiction than mental health problems. Although schizophrenia, bipolar disorder, Alzheimer's, and ADHD wreak more havoc on the life of the patient, their family, and their friends than does anxiety disorder, in most cases, the ability of this disorder to interfere with a "normal" life cannot and should not be ignored or downplayed. Treatment, whether by drug, talk, or other therapies can be beneficial and should be discussed with patients.

Not So Anonymous

ANXIETY

Although anxiety and insomnia are frequently discussed separately in psychopharmacology textbooks, these two problems often coexist and many of the drugs used to treat one are also used to treat the other. Each issue is discussed individually first and then together at the end of this chapter.

Anxiety may be the most common psychological issue in the United States today. War, a housing crisis, an economic meltdown, and many other stressors have a way of inducing anxiety. According to *Merriam-Webster's Medical Dictionary*, anxiety is defined as:

1: a painful or apprehensive uneasiness of mind usually over an impending or anticipated ill;

2: an abnormal and overwhelming sense of apprehension and fear often marked by physiological signs (as sweating, tension, and increased pulse), by doubt concerning the reality and nature of the threat, and by self-doubt about one's capacity to cope with it

Anxiety is normal and everyone experiences it with varying degrees of intensity throughout life. From an evolutionary perspective, it is an alarm that is supposed to protect a person from harm. But sometimes the level of anxiety and its symptoms are disproportionate to the actual danger and interfere with a person's ability to function. When this occurs, treatment—including drugs—may be needed to help the patient. There are several distinct anxiety disorder subtypes, based on the diagnostic criteria in the DSM-IV-TR (American Psychiatric Association, 2000), including: Panic Disorder with or without Agoraphobia, Agoraphobia without History of Panic Disorder, Specific Phobia, Social Phobia, Obsessive-Compulsive Disorder, Post-traumatic Stress Disorder, Acute Stress Disorder, Generalized Anxiety Disorder, Anxiety Disorder Due to a General Medical Condition, Substance-Induced Anxiety Disorder, and Anxiety Disorder Not Otherwise Specified.

Primary care physicians usually treat generalized anxiety disorder (GAD) symptomatically without ever applying specific diagnostic criteria (Stahl, 2008). Psychiatrists, on the other hand, seem more interested in GAD only insofar as it is a common comorbid condition in patients with the other "more severe" anxiety disorder subtypes or in those with major depressive disorder. GAD may be a comorbid factor in other nonpsychiatric medical disorders such as irritable bowel syndrome, asthma, cardiovascular disease, cancer, and chronic pain (Kessler et al., 2008; Roy-Byrne et al., 2008). GAD is a chronic disorder, with symptoms that wax and wane over years or decades of a patient's life (Moore & Jefferson, 2004).

PHARMACOTHERAPY OF ANXIETY

Beginning in the 1960s, anxiety was treated with the benzodiazepines and depression was treated with MAOIs or TCAs. This reflected a view that depression and anxiety were distinct entities. Moreover, all anxiety disorders were treated uniformly. It didn't matter whether the patient had a panic disorder, a social phobia, obsessive-compulsive disorder, or "merely" generalized anxiety disorder; all of these conditions were treated with a benzodiazepine (Tone, 2005). In the late 1970s and early 1980s, clinicians recognized that certain tricyclic antidepressants and MAO inhibitors were better than benzodiazepines for treating panic disorder and that clomipramine (Anafranil), a tricyclic antidepressant, was most effective for obsessive compulsive disorder (Nemeroff, 2003). The finding that antidepressants might be effective in treating certain forms of anxiety is consistent with the view that these patients may have mixed anxiety depression (MAD), in which the patient has both major depressive disorder (MDD) and generalized anxiety disorder (GAD).

In the 1990s, the selective serotonin reuptake inhibitors (SSRIs) began their ascent as a first-line treatment for essentially all anxiety disorder subtypes. Whether the newer antidepressants share this therapeutic efficacy is not yet settled. Venlafaxine XR (Effexor), however, has been found clinically effective in treating both mood disturbances in depression and anxiety in GAD. It is a broad spectrum psychotropic that can be used in both mood and anxiety disorders (Moore & Jefferson, 2004). In the past an SSRI could be used to treat both depression and anxiety disorder subtypes. If a patient had a major depressive disorder (MDD) and GAD, an antianxiety drug needed to be added.

Many drugs have been used to treat anxiety. The most common drug is self-administered and not prescribed. It is alcohol. The drugs prescribed to treat depression fall into one of three classes, depending on whether their mechanism involves the neurotransmitters 5-HT, NE, or gamma amino butyric acid (GABA) (Kirkwood & Melton, 2005).

5-HT Anxiolytics

The prototypical 5-HT$_{1A}$ (partial) agonist is buspirone (BuSpar). Although studies suggest that this drug is neither a powerful anxiolytic nor an efficient antidepressant, it offers certain advantages over the benzodiazepines in the treatment of anxiety. It does not interact with alcohol or other anxiolytic-sedative-hypnotic drugs, and it does not produce drug dependence or withdrawal symptoms with chronic use. These assets also make it an effective drug in patients with a prior history of drug and/or alcohol abuse. The major disadvantage, when compared to benzodiazepines, is a delay in clinical improvement, similar to what is seen when it is used for depression. This suggests that the clinical improvement seen with 5-HT$_{1A}$ agonists is due to adaptive changes, rather than to a direct action on their receptors.

Also, buspirone (BuSpar) might be considered first-line therapy for patients with chronic, persistent anxiety (GAD) and patients with substance abuse issues. It also may be useful in elderly patients because of the low incidence of drug interactions and because it is well tolerated (Stahl, 2008).

NE Anxiolytics

Anxiety symptoms associated with excessive sympathetic autonomic nervous system activity include tachycardia, tremor, sweating, and dilated pupils. An important noradrenergic pathway (Figure 6-1) in the brain, which may be overactive in anxious subjects, originates the locus ceruleus.

Assuming that excessive amounts of NE are released throughout the body and are producing the above symptoms, there are two NE receptor–based approaches to diminish these symptoms. The first approach decreases release of NE, via presynaptic NE autoreceptors (α_2) and the second blocks the appropriate postsynaptic receptors (β) for NE (Figure 6-2).

An effective anxiolytic that acts by stimulating presynaptic α_2 NE autoreceptors is clonidine (Catapres). Stimulating the α_2 autoreceptor decreases additional NE release and thus lowers the level of NE (in the synapse) that can act on postsynaptic receptors. Clonidine is also used to treat hypertension and the withdrawal symptoms

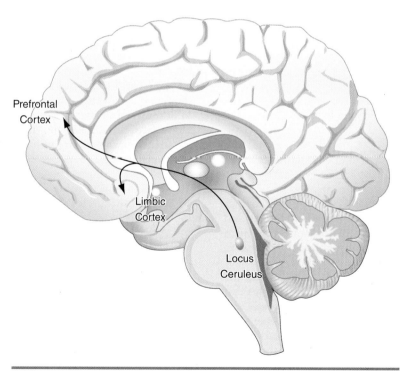

FIGURE 6-1 Brain norepinephrine (NE) pathways originating in the locus ceruleus, terminating in the prefrontal cortex and the limbic system.

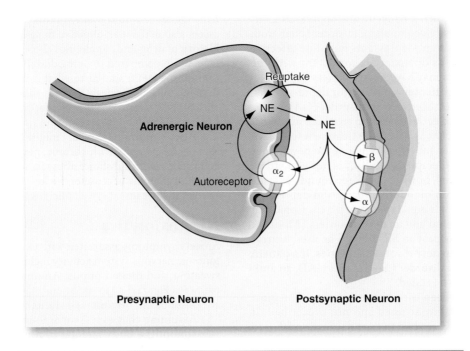

FIGURE 6-2 Adrenergic neurons and receptors. When norepinephrine (NE) is released by adrenergic neurons, it can act postsynaptically on α or β receptors or presynaptically on α₂ receptors, to regulate release of additional NE. Higher levels of NE acting on these presynaptic autoreceptors decrease additional release of NE.

from a number of addictive substances, including alcohol, barbiturates, opioids, and benzodiazepines.

Many of the above autonomic signs of anxiety are mediated by beta adrenoceptors and can be reduced by giving the patient a beta blocker, such as propranolol (Inderal). Both clonidine and propranolol are particularly effective at blocking the noradrenergic signs of anxiety including tachycardia, dilated pupils, sweating, and tremor, although neither drug works as well on the subjective and emotional aspects of anxiety. The NE anxiolytics may be the drugs of choice for social phobias.

GABA Anxiolytics

GABA is the most important and abundant inhibitory neurotransmitter in the brain. GABA acts on two postsynaptic receptors, GABA$_A$ and GABA$_B$ receptors. It is known that the GABA$_A$ receptor mediates a wide range of CNS activities and is the site of action for benzodiazepines, barbiturates, and alcohol (behavioral effects). GABA$_B$ receptors are involved in the muscle-relaxing action of baclofen but do not appear to play a role in anxiety or insomnia.

The GABA$_A$ receptor (Figure 6-3) is different from the other receptors that have been discussed thus far. Drugs that act via this receptor do not bind to the receptor at the GABA binding site. The GABA$_A$ receptor complex has multiple binding sites, including one for GABA, one for benzodiazepines, and yet another for barbiturates (and perhaps a fourth for ethanol) (Charney, Mihic, & Harris, 2006).

When GABA binds to its receptor, it opens chloride (Cl$^-$) channels, allowing the negatively charged ion to slowly enter the cell. This hyperpolarizes the cell, making it more difficult for the cell to trigger an action potential. By definition, this makes GABA an inhibitory neurotransmitter. When benzodiazepines bind to the secondary binding sites, they facilitate GABA binding and Cl$^-$ floods into the cell, making it still more difficult to trigger action potentials. This activity is what makes these drugs CNS depressants and what makes them effective as anxiolytics, sedative-hypnotics, and muscle relaxants.

The barbiturates are not used to treat anxiety because they are only effective at reducing anxiety at hypnotic doses. In other words, patients are not functional while under the influence of barbiturates; they fall asleep.

Benzodiazepines are used clinically to treat both anxiety and sleep disorders (Table 6-1). All benzodiazepines can be used to control seizures, although only a few are marketed for this purpose. Some benzodiazepines (but not all) also cause muscle relaxation. Diazepam (Valium) is one such drug.

A troubling side effect of many benzodiazepines is amnesia, which is also mediated by these receptors. One benzodiazepine, flunitrazepam (Rohypnol; not approved by the FDA), has an unsavory reputation. It is the so-called "date rape" drug (Charney et al., 2006). Because of its extremely high potency it can be added to alcoholic beverages without altering the taste, making it virtually undetectable by anyone consuming it. It profoundly affects the memory of the user ("victim" is a more appropriate term) for several hours after consumption. The user may be awake and communicative but has no memory of what happened after consuming the drug.

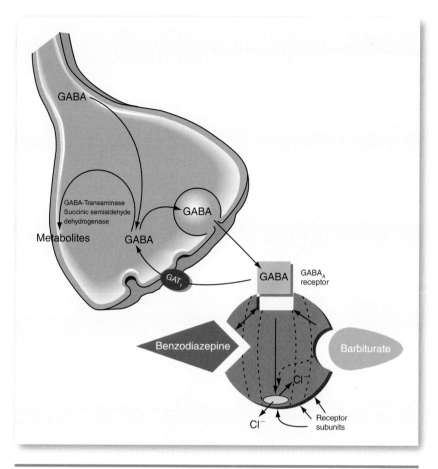

FIGURE 6-3 GABA receptor complex with binding sites for GABA, barbiturates (BARB), and benzodiazepines (BENZO).

TABLE 6-1 Common Benzodiazepines

GENERIC	TRADE	HALF-LIFE (HR)	CLINICAL USES
Triazolam	Halcion	2-6	Hypnosis
Temazepam	Restoril	5-20	Hypnosis
Oxazepam	Serax	6-24	Anxiety
Alprazolam	Xanax	6-20	Anxiety ± depression
Chlordiazepoxide	Librium	7-46	Anxiety
Lorazepam	Ativan	9-22	Anxiety
Estazolam	Prosom	10-24	Hypnosis
Diazepam	Valium	14-90	Anxiety
Quazepam	Doral	30-100	Hypnosis
Clorazepate	Tranxene	30-200	Anxiety
Prazepam	Centrax	30-200	Anxiety
Halazepam	Paxipam	30-200	Anxiety
Flurazepam	Dalmane	90-200	Hypnosis

INSOMNIA

Insomnia (Latin for "no sleep") can have many causes, although for most people it is only an occasional problem. Sometimes insomnia should be treated with drugs and other times, not. People's perception of their own sleep disturbances may be different from reality, and the spate of commercials on television, radio, or print media only reinforce these beliefs. According to the 2009 Sleep in America™ Poll conducted by the National Sleep Foundation, over 40% of the US population felt they were not getting enough sleep, over 40% slept less than six hours per night (on weeknights), 43% used a sleep-aid more than once per week, and 25% were told by a doctor that they had a sleep disorder (National Sleep Foundation, 2009). In most cases, simple solutions, such as improved "sleep hygiene," can improve the situation. Better sleep hygiene includes keeping regular sleep/wake hours, avoiding daytime naps, not using the bed for work activities, and skipping caffeinated beverages after the dinner hour. Sleep problems can have a medical basis (e.g., sleep apnea, restless legs syndrome), and can be due to depression. As such, treatment of the underlying condition may resolve the sleep disturbance. Difficulty sleeping may also be a result of a decreased need for sleep with aging (Bliwise, 2000).

When pharmacological measures are deemed necessary, treatment is rarely recommended beyond a few days for transient insomnia (e.g., jet-lag), a few weeks for short-term insomnia (e.g., divorce, family illness, or death), or, at most, a few months (one night in three) for long-term insomnia. However, because of the debilitating nature of this complaint—it is not a disease—for some people, the relative safety of the newer drugs and the slow rate of tolerance development may allow patients to take some of these drugs for longer periods.

PHARMACOLOGIC MANAGEMENT OF INSOMNIA

Using alcohol to self-medicate for sleep difficulties dates back to early human civilization. With the development of barbiturates in the early twentieth century the modern medical age of insomnia management truly began. Two drugs in particular, secobarbital (Seconal) and pentobarbital (Nembutal), were the mainstays for treating sleep problems until the mid-1960s when the benzodiazepines were discovered and quickly replaced the barbiturates as the drugs of choice for sleep problems (and anxiety) (Charney et al., 2006).

Although the barbiturates were unquestionably effective, they had two challenging characteristics. Barbiturates are a notorious group of drugs that induce (stimulate) hepatic drug-metabolizing enzymes (CYP) with chronic usage. Because of this, prescribers often had to raise the dose of other drugs the patient might be taking, and then reduce them when the patient went off of the barbiturate. Polypharmacy, in other words, is a problem if one of the drugs is a barbiturate.

Second, with long-term use, the therapeutic index of barbiturates gets lower and lower, so that, over time, the therapeutic dose begins to approach the lethal dose. Even as late as the 1980s the most common form of lethal prescription drug overdoses in the United States occurred with barbiturates.

With benzodiazepines, neither of these problems is seen. Polypharmacy issues occur only with CNS depressants, such as opioids and alcohol, for example. Moreover, the therapeutic index for benzodiazepines is quite high and remains so over the duration of treatment. It is clear that benzodiazepines had distinct practical advantages over barbiturates in treating insomnia.

Today, another group of drugs has replaced the benzodiazepines as first-line therapy for insomnia. These are the non-benzodiazepine benzodiazepine (BZ)-receptor agonists (Charney et al., 2006). These drugs bind to the BZ receptor, but they do not fit the precise chemical structure to be classified as a benzodiazepine. The classes of drugs commonly used today to treat insomnia include the BZs, the non-BZ BZ-receptor agonists (NBBAs), antidepressants, over-the-counter (OTC) drugs, and a miscellaneous drug or two.

Benzodiazepines

The mechanism of action of the benzodiazepines for treating insomnia is the same as the mechanism for their anxiolytic actions. That is, they act on the BZ-receptor-binding site on the $GABA_A$ receptor complex in several areas of the brain. All benzodiazepines are anxiolytic-sedative-hypnotics. In their clinical use differences among the drugs have had more to do with their duration of action than to their mechanism of action (i.e., for their pharmacokinetic vs. pharmacodynamic characteristics). The BZs may be classified as rapid-onset and short-acting (e.g., triazolam—Halcion); delayed-onset and intermediate-acting (e.g., temazepam—Restoril); or rapid-onset and long-acting (flurazepam—Dalmane). When patients have sleep problems, they generally have one of two complaints; difficulty falling asleep (sleep onset) or remaining asleep (frequent or early awakening). Some patients have both complaints and others describe ongoing daytime anxiety as well.

BZs that are rapid-onset and short-acting are effective for sleep onset issues, but are less effective for early awakening problems. In fact, they may worsen this problem. For delayed-onset, intermediate-acting drugs, the reverse is often the case, and the drugs do little if the patient's main complaint is getting to sleep. Although rapid-onset, long-acting drugs are effective for both types of insomnia, the persistence of effect into the daytime hours may make them unsuitable for many patients, but these may be the BZ drugs of choice if the patient has daytime anxiety issues.

Non-benzodiazepine Benzodiazepine Agonists (NBBAs)

Currently there are three drugs sold in the United States that fit the description of non-benzodiazepine benzodiazepine agonists (NBBAs). These are zolpidem (Ambien and Ambien CR), zaleplon (Sonata), and eszopiclone (Lunesta), three of the most heavily advertised drugs marketed today. These drugs all bind to a single subtype of the benzodiazepine receptor. The only thing that drugs binding to this receptor do is improve sleep; they are not anxiolytic or anticonvulsant and they do not affect memory (see next paragraph, however),

TABLE 6-2 Comparison of BZs and NBBAs

	BENZODIAZEPINE RECEPTOR	
	OMEGA 1	OMEGA 2
Benzodiazepines	Yes	Yes
Non-benzodiazepine benzodiazepine agonists	Yes	No
Effect	Sleep	Anxiety, seizures, memory

© Delmar/Cengage Learning

a common problem with benzodiazepines. They also have little if any abuse potential and little efficacy is lost over time (no tolerance).

A series of media (not medical) reports have emerged in the few years of unusual patient behaviors while under the influence of zolpidem (Ambien). These include sleep-walking, sleep-driving ("Your honor, please understand, the drug caused the accident. I don't remember anything after I took the Ambien."), sleep-gambling, and sleep-binging. The claims have not been scientifically validated; it is not clear if they occur with other NBBAs, and it is not known what, if any, other drugs these people were taking when they experienced these side effects. However, it is important that prescribers discuss this concern with patients who are taking these drugs.

Today, the NBBAs are the drugs of choice for treating insomnia. While these drugs have a lower abuse potential than the benzodiazepines, they are still DEA controlled substances and can only be prescribed by persons who are DEA licensed.

The next groups of drugs have no abuse potential, do not require a DEA license, and some are sold over the counter.

Antidepressants for Insomnia

Several antidepressants, particularly the tricyclics, cause drowsiness as an adverse effect when they are used to treat depression. While they have lost favor as first-line therapy for depression, they have seen resurgence for other purposes, including insomnia. The mechanism for this action is blockade of histaminergic (H_1) and muscarinic-cholinergic (M) receptors in the brain and is independent of their antidepressant action, as discussed in Chapter 2.

Over-the-Counter (OTC) Sleep Aids

Almost all OTC sleep aids contain an antihistamine, most often diphenhydramine, which is the active ingredient in the allergy medication Benadryl. Although diphenhydramine is an effective allergy drug, it frequently causes daytime drowsiness, which limits its use. Taken at bedtime, however, this is an asset not a liability. Any drug with a "PM" in its trade name (Tylenol PM, Advil PM) contains diphenhydramine. The combination

of an antihistamine (H_1 receptor antagonist) and an analgesic may help with sleep.

Melatonin-based Drugs

The suprachiasmatic nucleus (SCN) in the brain is known as the body's "master clock." It regulates 24-hour, or circadian rhythms, including the sleep-wake cycle. The key neurotransmitter in the SCN is melatonin. Ramelteon (Rozerem) is an agonist at melatonin receptors in the SCN (Miyamoto, 2009; Reynoldson, Elliott, & Nelson, 2008). Overall adverse events (most commonly headache) occur at rates generally comparable to placebo and there is no evidence of physical dependence or abuse potential. Also, unlike many other sleep medications, ramelteon does not affect motor function or cognition (Reynoldson et al., 2008), and it has been approved by the FDA for long-term use in adults.

Dietary Supplements

Several dietary supplements and herbs are marketed to improve sleep health (not to treat insomnia). These include melatonin, valerian root, hops, chamomile, and lemon balm (NIH—Office of Dietary Supplements). When melatonin is used in this way, patients (and prescribers) should be aware that the FDA does not regulate it for safety or efficacy. Furthermore, there is significant brand-to-brand variation in dosages (2 to 3 mg vs. natural levels in the body of 0.1 to 0.3 mg). Additionally, there is no consensus on what is the effective dose of melatonin for sleep, and there is evidence that doses above 1 mg may actually disturb sleep.

EVOLVING DRUG OPTIONS

It was not until the 1960s that truly safe, effective anxiolytic–sedative–hypnotics—the benzodiazepines—were discovered. Later, researchers and clinicians came to recognize that other psychoactive drugs were also effective in treating anxiety. Knowing the type of anxiety the patient is experiencing—GAD, social anxiety disorder, panic disorder, etc.—allows clinicians to choose drugs with mechanisms of action that are targeted to specific anxiety symptoms. For some types of anxiety, drugs whose mechanism of action involves serotonin work best. With other types of anxiety, a norepinephrine-based mechanism is preferable, and with still others drugs acting via GABA are ideal. It's nice to have choices and options.

For insomnia, alcohol begat barbiturates, which begat benzodiazepines, which begat non-benzodiazepine benzodiazepine agonists, today's drugs of choice for sleep disorders. The shift has been from a generalized CNS depressant (alcohol) to a class of drugs (barbiturates) that were more selective in their action on the brain. This then led to drugs (benzodiazepines) that had fewer drug interactions and a better safety record. Today, the drugs for insomnia (NBBAs) are far more specific than anything in the past. They improve sleep and do little else (except perhaps provide an excuse for a midnight Twinkie jag). They have little abuse potential and tolerance develops quite slowly.

REVIEW QUESTIONS

Match each of the following drugs with the neurotransmitter believed responsible for its mechanism of action

1. Buspirone (BuSpar)   a. 5-HT
2. Diazepam (Valium)   b. Melatonin
3. Propranolol (Inderal)   c. Norepinephrine
4. Ramelteon (Rozerem)   d. GABA

5. Which sedative/anxiolytic drug(s) listed below bind(s) to a site on the receptor complex other than where the neurotransmitter GABA binds?
   a. Triazolam (Halcion)
   b. Alprazolam (Xanax)
   c. Zolpidem (Ambien)
   d. All of the above

6. What clinical condition(s) is zaleplon (Sonata) used to treat?
   a. Anxiety
   b. Insomnia
   c. Epilepsy
   d. All of the above

7. Thomas Kruz is a patient who is having difficulty sleeping but he refuses to use "Western medicine" drugs. Which of the following dietary supplements/herbs might be used to help improve his sleep?
   a. Bromelain
   b. Ginkgo biloba
   c. Valerian root
   d. Yohimbe

8. Which of the following facts about barbiturates is not true?
   a. Barbiturates are inducers of cytochrome P450 (CYP) enzymes.
   b. With long-tem use, the therapeutic index (LD50 ÷ ED50) of barbiturates declines.
   c. When used alone (i.e., no polypharmacy), high doses of barbiturates can cause respiratory and cardiovascular system depression.
   d. Low doses (i.e., less than sedating) of barbiturates are anxiolytic.

9. What is the proposed mechanism of action for beta-blockers such as propranolol (Inderal) in treating anxiety?
   a. 5-HT_{2A} agonist
   b. Dopamine receptor antagonist
   c. $GABA_A$ receptor modulator
   d. Beta adrenergic receptor blocker

10. What class of drugs are drugs are commonly used in over-the-counter sleep aids?
    a. Antihistamines
    b. Beta blockers
    c. Benzodiazepines
    d. NMDA antagonists

REFERENCES

American Psychiatric Association. (2000). *Diagnostic and statistical manual of mental disorders: DSM-IV-TR.* (4th ed.) Washington, DC: American Psychiatric Association.

Bliwise, D. L. (Ed.). (2000). *Normal aging* (3rd ed.). Philadelphia: W. B. Saunders.

Charney, D. S., Mihic, S. J., & Harris, R. A. (2006). Hypnotics and sedatives. In L. L. Brunton, J. S. Lazo, & K. L. Parker (Eds.), *Goodman & Gilman's the pharmacological basis of therapeutics* (11th ed.). New York: McGraw-Hill.

Kessler, R. C., Gruber, M., Hettema, J. M., Hwang, I., Sampson, N., & Yonkers, K. A. (2008). Co-morbid major depression and generalized anxiety disorders in the National Comorbidity Survey follow-up. *Psychological Medicine, 38*(3), 365–374.

Kirkwood, C. K., & Melton, S. T. (2005). Anxiety disorders I; generalized anxiety, panic, and social anxiety disorders. In J. T. DiPiro, R. L. Talbert, G. C. Yee, G. R. Matzke, & B. G. Wells (Eds.), *Pharmacotherapy: A pathophysiologic approach* (6th ed.) (pp. 1285–1305). New York: McGraw-Hill Medical.

Miyamoto, M. (2009). Pharmacology of ramelteon, a selective MT1/MT2 receptor agonist: A novel therapeutic drug for sleep disorders. *CNS Neuroscience & Therapeutics, 15*(1), 32–51.

Moore, D. P., & Jefferson, J. W. (2004). Generalized anxiety disorder. *Moore & Jefferson: Handbook of medical psychiatry* (2nd ed.). St. Louis, Mo: Mosby.

National Sleep Foundation. *Sleep in America Poll, 2009.* Retrieved 1/23/2010, from http://www.sleepfoundation.org/article/sleep-america-polls/2009-health-and-safety.

Nemeroff, C. B. (2003). Anxiolytics: Past, present, and future agents. *Journal of Clinical Psychiatry, 64*(Suppl 3), 3–6.

NIH—Office of Dietary Supplements. *Dietary supplement fact sheets.* Retrieved 5/13/2009, from http://dietary-supplements.info.nih.gov/Health_Information/Information_About_Individual_Dietary_Supplements.aspx

Reynoldson, J. N., Elliott, E., Sr., & Nelson, L. A. (2008). Ramelteon: A novel approach in the treatment of insomnia. *Annals of Pharmacotherapy, 42*(9), 1262–1271.

Roy-Byrne, P. P., Davidson, K. W., Kessler, R. C., Asmundson, G. J., Goodwin, R. D., Kubzansky, L., et al. (2008). Anxiety disorders and comorbid medical illness. *General Hospital Psychiatry, 30*(3), 208–225.

Stahl, S. M. (2008). *Stahl's essential psychopharmacology: Neuroscientific basis and practical applications* (3rd ed.). New York: Cambridge University Press.

Tone, A. (2005). Listening to the past: History, psychiatry, and anxiety. *Canadian Journal of Psychiatry—Revue Canadienne De Psychiatrie, 50*(7), 373–380.

CHAPTER 7

Neurobiology of Addiction

"What a crazy world we live in! Trying to treat addiction as a legal problem, and trying to treat criminal misbehaviors using guns as a medical problem! Beam me up, Scotty. Ain't no intelligent life down here."

JULIE COCHRANE

GETTING PERSONAL

I was a typical college student. I had my grades in order and a bright future in the horizon. I smoked pot to mellow out after class and drank to enjoy the weekends. Neither drug got out of hand and I never craved or needed either to deal with any sort of problem. Unfortunately, I came across one drug that really made me feel good and I never forgot that amazing feeling and euphoria, something neither pot nor alcohol ever gave me. The drug was hydrocodone (Vicodin), which is a narcotic pain medication.

In my later years of college, I occasionally came across a "pharmy," as we called the drug, and I never sought or took one for more than a day or two. Following college I got a very lucrative job in Los Angeles and life was great. I had my life in order, a great future ahead of me and I felt no need for any drug. Unfortunately, the bubble burst and within a year period my stepmother (since I was 2 years old) died from cancer, my remaining grandparents died, I lost my

job and apartment in Los Angeles, broke up with my girlfriend, and was forced to move home. At this point I was grief stricken. I had nowhere to turn and I gave in to narcotics, which gave me so much pleasure and made me forget at least for a while all that I had lost. I had an unlimited access to oxycontin through friends and plenty of leftover pain medication from my stepmother's bout with cancer. At first I took the drugs to mellow out at night, but as the months passed I needed more and more to get high and then I always needed it. From the time I woke up to until I went to bed I was high.
I tried to cut back or quit many times, but the withdrawal symptoms were overwhelming. I finally realized that I was so addicted I had to take pain medication just to feel normal. I hit rock bottom realizing I had lied, stolen, and blown through most of my money. After almost a year of hardcore abuse, I finally confessed to my family of my addiction and abuse.

With my family's encouragement I entered a treatment program, one that dealt with underlying mental health issues as well as my addiction. As bad as I had it, I saw in others how much worse it could get and swore that it would never happen to me again.
I have many various support groups, including my family and friends, AA, as well as my doctors. I am currently on a medication called suboxone, which completely prevents any withdrawal symptoms and helps block cravings and urges. I have been sober and in recovery for over 10 months and have started to become successful again.

Anonymous

STATISTICS

According to the National Institute on Drug Abuse (2009), drug addiction is "a disease that is characterized by compulsive drug seeking and use, despite harmful consequences. It is considered a brain disease because drugs change the brain—they change its structure and how it works. These brain changes can be long lasting, and can lead to the harmful behaviors seen in people who abuse drugs."

Surprisingly, the *Diagnostic and Statistical Manual of Mental Disorders*, Text Revision, Fourth Edition (American Psychiatric Association, 2000), the central document for American mental health providers on the classification of psychiatric disorders, does not classify addiction in its Listing of DSM-IV-TR Diagnoses and Codes or anywhere else. Does this imply that drug addiction is a disease but not a psychiatric disorder? The truth is, the editors who periodically update the DSM now use the terms "substance use disorder" or "substance dependence and substance abuse" instead of "drug addiction" to describe the same behaviors (Tables 7-1 and 7-2). In the future don't be surprised if the term *addiction* returns to the APA lexicon once the DSM-V is eventually released (Fainsinger, Thai, Frank, & Fergusson, 2006; O'Brien, Volkow, & Li, 2006).

What are some of the facts about substance abuse from the National Survey on Drug Use and Health (NSDUH), which is published annually by the Substance Abuse and Mental Health Services Administration (SAMHSA)? In SAMHSA's 2008 report (Office of Applied Studies, 2009) 20.1 million Americans at least 12 years of age have used illicit drugs in the previous month. These drugs include marijuana/hashish, cocaine, heroin, hallucinogens, inhalants, and prescription psychotherapeutics that are used nontherapeutically. The data indicate that within a given month 8% of the U.S. population uses illicit drugs—not including alcohol or tobacco products. SAMHSA estimates that 6.2 million people use prescription psychotherapeutic agents (predominantly opioids) for nonmedical reasons. Keep in mind, that is not lifetime prevalence, just recent and current use.

In 2008 about 129 million (51.6%) Americans, age 12 years or older, used alcohol within the previous 30 days and 58.1 million participated in binge drinking (having five or more drinks on the same occasion on at least 1 day in the 30 days prior to the survey). Fortunately, tobacco use in this age group declined from 30.4% of the population in 2002 to 28.4% in 2008. Based on the criteria in DSM-IV (Tables 7-1 and 7-2), about 22.2 million people (9%) 12 years of age or older had a substance use disorder in 2008. Of these, 3.1 million were classified with a substance use disorder of both alcohol and illicit drugs, 3.9 million were dependent on or abused illicit drugs but not alcohol, and 15.2 million were dependent on or abused alcohol but not illicit drugs.

According to the 2008 SAMHSA report, the incidence of substance use disorders among adults 18 years of age or older is about three times higher in people with serious mental illness (SMI) than in those without it (25.2% vs. 8.3%). SMI "is defined in Public Law 102-321 as persons aged 18 or older who currently or at any time in the past year have had a diagnosable mental, behavioral, or emotional disorder (excluding developmental and substance use disorders) of sufficient duration to meet diagnostic criteria specified within DSM-IV that has resulted in functional impairment, which substantially interferes with or limits one or more major life activities," as noted in the 2008 National Survey on Drug Use and Health. Similarly, adults who had a major depressive episode in the

TABLE 7-1 DSM-IV-TR Diagnostic Criteria for Substance Dependence

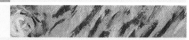

The DSM-IV defines the diagnostic criteria for substance dependence as a maladaptive pattern of substance use, leading to clinically significant impairment or distress, as manifested by three or more of the following, occurring at any time in the same 12-month period:

1. Tolerance, as defined by either of the following:

   a. The need for markedly increased amounts of the substance to achieve intoxication or desired effect.

   b. Markedly diminished effect with continued use of the same amount of the substance.

2. Withdrawal, as manifested by either of the following:

   a. The characteristic withdrawal syndrome for the substance.

   b. The same (or closely related) substance is taken to relieve or avoid withdrawal symptoms.

3. Taking the substance often in larger amounts or over a longer period than was intended.

4. A persistent desire or unsuccessful efforts to cut down or control substance use.

5. Spending a great deal of time in activities necessary to obtain or use the substance or to recover from its effects.

6. Giving up social, occupational, or recreational activities because of substance use.

7. Continuing the substance use with the knowledge that it is causing or exacerbating a persistent or recurrent physical or psychological problem.

Source: Reprinted with permission from the *Diagnostic and Statistical Manual of Mental Disorders,* Fourth Edition, Text Revision. Copyright 2000 American Psychiatric Association.

© Delmar/Cengage Learning

TABLE 7-2 DSM-IV-TR Diagnostic Criteria for Substance Abuse

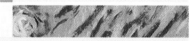

The DSM-IV defines the diagnostic criteria for substance abuse as a maladaptive pattern of substance use leading to clinically significant impairment or distress, as manifested by one or more of the following, occurring within a 12-month period:

1. Recurrent substance use resulting in a failure to fulfill major role obligations at work, school, or home (e.g., repeated absences or poor work performance related to substance use; substance-related absences, suspensions, or expulsions from school; neglect of children or household).

2. Recurrent substance use in situations in which it is physically hazardous (e.g., driving an automobile or operating a machine when impaired by substance use).

3. Recurrent substance-related legal problems (e.g., arrests for substance-related disorderly conduct).

4. Continued substance use despite having persistent or recurrent social or interpersonal problems caused or exacerbated by the effects of the substance (e.g., arguments with spouse about consequences of intoxication, physical fights).

Source: Reprinted with permission from the *Diagnostic and Statistical Manual of Mental Disorders,* Fourth Edition, Text Revision. Copyright 2000, American Psychiatric Association.

© Delmar/Cengage Learning

previous year were about twice as likely to have a substance use disorder than those without a major depressive episode (27.2% vs. 13.0%).

Of the 2.5 million individuals who had both SMI and a substance use disorder, only 11.4% received both mental health care and substance use treatment in a specialty clinic, whereas 45.2% received only mental health care, and 3.7% were treated only in a specialty substance use program. As importantly, 39.5% received no treatment whatsoever. Thus, it appears that the majority of people with a dual diagnosis mental-health/substance-use disorder are not getting professional help for both problems. More often than not, patients and mental health professionals are trying to resolve the problems sequentially rather than concurrently. This may help explain the relatively high rate of treatment failure rate in addiction (National Institutes of Health, 2009).

ADDICTION

Every day new statistics about the problem of drug abuse and addiction appear in newspapers, television, radio, and on the Internet. The breadth of this subject matter is simply too expansive to address in one chapter of one book. Thus, this chapter focuses on a few drugs and only within certain parameters. The key drug classes examined include opioids, anxiolytic-sedative-hypnotics, psychostimulants, and a few additional drugs (marijuana and alcohol). The parameters include the drugs' mechanisms of action, the sites of action in the brain, (potential) clinical utility, why the drugs may be abused, and what treatments are available to treat addiction.

TERMS

While many of the words used throughout this chapter—*narcotic*, to begin with—are common terms, they may have astonishingly different meanings to different audiences. Thus, the next few paragraphs will cover a few terms to clarify their intent and implications.

NARCOTIC

What, for example, does the word *narcotic* mean? For professionals involved in health care it is synonymous with opiate or opioid, but in law enforcement it may imply something entirely different. Examples of a "narcotic drug" listed in Section 802 of the United States Controlled Substances Act (U.S. Department of Justice, Drug Enforcement Administration), include "[o]pium, opiates, derivatives of opium . . ." and "[c]ocaine, its salts, optical and geometric isomers, and salts of isomers." A nurse, a physician, a pharmacist, or anyone else in health care would never identify cocaine as a narcotic. The most unmistakable and least ambiguous term for natural or synthetic drugs with morphine-like properties is *opioid*, leaving no confusion or doubt that the term means the same thing to everyone.

DRUG DEPENDENCE

Drug dependence is a state in which the use of a drug is necessary for either the physical or psychological well-being of the user. In physical/physiological dependence, some as yet unknown changes take place at the cellular level, accompanied by the appearance of a characteristic withdrawal syndrome upon rapid termination of drug use. Depending on the drug and the level of dependence, withdrawal may manifest as increased heart rate and blood pressure, sweating, muscle cramping, tremors or, more seriously, as confusion, hallucinations, and potentially lethal seizures.

Not all dependence, however, is physical. Some users may express only psychological signs and symptoms. When people who are psychologically dependent lose access to their drug of choice, they may be overcome with a sense of impending doom or peril, even though there is no clearly measurable withdrawal syndrome or tolerance to the drug when it is actually removed (which might occur someone is confined in a hospital or jail).

It is important to recognize that physical dependence may occur with drugs that have no pleasurable effects and are not abused. For example, when certain antihypertensive drugs—beta blockers, for example—are used for extended periods, precipitous discontinuation can be potentially lethal. Other drugs, such as steroids, induce physiological changes in the patient and dosage must be tapered during discontinuation to avoid serious adverse effects. In an odd sort of way, this too is a form of physical dependence, although it may not be identified as such.

Physical dependence is not the same thing as addiction. Cancer patients often become physically dependent on opioids when these drugs are used for extended periods for pain management. During remission these patients must be weaned off of the drug to avoid withdrawal. However, by no stretch of the imagination are they considered to be drug addicts. Surprisingly (or not surprisingly), cancer patients or their family and friends may worry about addiction, which may lead patients to avoid the use of opioids—resulting in inadequate pain control.

TOLERANCE

Tolerance occurs when certain drugs are taken repeatedly and they become less effective over time. Another way of stating this is: in order to achieve the same pharmacological effect of a drug over time the dose must be escalated. Tolerance does not occur equally to all drugs (more profound for opioids than stimulants) or even at the same rate for different actions (more rapid tolerance to the analgesic than to the constipating action of opioids) in the same patient. Also, if people are tolerant to one drug in a class they are also tolerant to other drugs in that same class. For example, in the event of an injury heroin abusers require higher doses of morphine—or other opioids—for pain. Similarly, alcoholics often need significantly higher doses of benzodiazepines or barbiturates than the nonalcoholic patient to manage anxiety, sleep, or epilepsy.

PSYCHOACTIVE DRUGS

Although all drugs of abuse are psychoactive (i.e., they affect behavior), not all psychoactive drugs are abused. These are not synonymous terms. Opioids, benzodiazepines, and amphetamines are often abused, but it is unlikely that anyone is abusing chlorpromazine, fluoxetine, or St. John's wort. Why are some psychoactive drugs abused and others are not?

The answer to this question lies with Burrhus Frederic (B. F.) Skinner. His basic theory of human and animal behavior (1938) was built on the truism that "a behavior followed by a reinforcing stimulus results in an increased probability of that behavior occurring in the future." If a drug has pleasurable actions (euphoria), it is more likely to be taken again (and again and again) than a drug that has no such effect or one that produces dysphoria. A key element of abuse, therefore, is some kind of pleasurable sensation.

DRUG ABUSE

It might be surprising to know that *drug abuse* is not a pharmacological term or concept; rather, it is a sociological term. It is society, not health care, that defines the parameters of abuse. For example, the occasional consumption of an alcoholic beverage by someone over 21 years old is generally not considered drug abuse. Yet, taking an opioid, a benzodiazepine, or a stimulant, or inhaling marijuana for nonmedical reasons is considered to be drug abuse by the legal system and society, despite the fact that these drugs do not cause long-term permanent damage to brain tissue but damage does occur with ethanol, which is legal.

While society can change within years, physiology does not. Advertisements for drugs in the late 1800s and early 1900s included heroin for cough relief and cocaine tooth drops. In fact, the early formula for Coca-Cola had trace amounts of cocaine, when cocaine was the active ingredient to relieve exhaustion. It may be hard to believe but amphetamine (Benzedrine inhaler) was sold over-the-counter in the United States until the early 1950s.

Even today, the definition of drug abuse is shifting. In some states a patient may be arrested for "medical use" of marijuana, while in others it is no longer a crime, even though it is a DEA Schedule I[1] drug. It appears that the list of states legalizing or decriminalizing (medical) marijuana use is growing. Does the marijuana of today have a different mechanism of action than it did a few years ago? Is it less toxic or healthier than it was at the millennium? No. The drug hasn't changed, but society has.

OPIOIDS, ANXIOLYTICS, AND STIMULANTS

The remainder of this chapter covers a limited number of drugs in detail, while others receive only brief attention. The focus is on drugs that are prescribed clinically, which include opioids, anxiolytics, and stimulants. The recreational drugs such as ethanol and marijuana are also covered. There is no treatise on LSD (Acid, Mellow Yellow), MDMA (Ecstasy, XTC, E, X, Beans, Adams), ketamine (Special K, Vitamin K, K), or dextromethorphan (DXM, CCC, Triple C, Skittles, Robo). There are too many drugs to cover in this brief survey.

OPIOIDS

Opioids are drugs that have morphine-like analgesic properties. At one time all drugs in this class were extracted directly from the opium poppy, *Papaver* (Greek for "poppy") *somniferum* (Latin for "I bring sleep"). The opium poppy was first cultivated circa 3400 BCE, in lower Mesopotamia. The Sumerians referred to it as the "joy plant" and would soon pass along the plant and share its euphoric effects with the Assyrians, who began cultivating it and distributing their knowledge and plants to the Babylonians and then the Egyptians. Thomas Sydenham (1624–1689), an Oxford-educated English physician, eloquently articulated, "Among the remedies which it has pleased the Almighty God to give to man to relieve his sufferings, none is so universal and efficacious as opium."

The German pharmacist Wilhelm Sertürner indentified the principal active ingredient in the opium poppy in 1805 and named it *morphium* (later morphine), after Morpheus, the Greek god of dreams. Widespread use followed by abuse did not occur in the United States until the mid-to-late 1800s, a time when the nation was divided by the Civil War.

The invention of the hypodermic syringe, the easy availability of opium (brought into the country by migrant Chinese railroad laborers and easily converted to morphine), and the presence of a large number of people (especially soldiers) in a great deal of pain (and, interestingly, unbearably bored between battles), set the groundwork for morphine's entry as a drug of abuse into American society. In 1866 Secretary of War Edwin Stanton reported that the Union Army issued 10 million opium pills, close to 3 million ounces of laudanum and paregoric, and almost 30,000 ounces of morphine sulfate to its soldiers during the Civil War.

Just as veterans coming home from Iraq and Afghanistan today return with post-traumatic stress disorder (PTSD), those returning home from the Civil War had their own distinctive disorder, know colloquially as Soldier's Disease. Actually, it was an opioid addiction that was accidentally acquired as a wartime memento. With the war finally over, the government in Washington was unsure about what to do with all the returning veterans on both sides who had become dependent on or addicted to morphine. It has been estimated[2] that about 400,000 Civil War veterans were afflicted with Soldier's Disease.

Recognizing the dark side of morphine, several drug manufacturers began to seek a non-addictive form of the morphine. German scientists at Bayer methodically manipulated morphine's molecular structure to create a drug they were sure would not have this problem and could, in fact, be used to combat morphine addiction. It was, by far, Bayer's best-selling brand of all time, marketed under the name Heroin (as it was thought to be the hero in medicine). Sometimes, even the best of intentions don't work out as planned[3].

Mechanism of Action

Since discovering both the benefits and the dangers of opium in pain control, scientists throughout the world have sought the Holy Grail of pharmacology (Corbett, Henderson, McKnight, & Paterson, 2006), a drug with the analgesic efficacy of morphine without its troubling adverse effects (sedation, respiratory depression, constipation, and high abuse potential). The hunt continues for this elusive and potentially miraculous drug, although researchers may now be closer to finding it as a result of over 200 years of daunting investigation. This is at least partly due to a better understanding of how opioids work.

The proposal that most drugs work via receptors is about a century old, but specific receptors for opioids were not definitively identified until the early 1970s (Pert & Snyder, 1973). Soon after that initial report, three distinct opioid receptor subtypes (μ, κ, and δ—renamed MOP, KOP, and DOP, respectively—Table 7-3) were identified. In 2000 the opioid receptor for nociceptin (NOP) was identified (Mollereau & Mouledous, 2000). Again, the hope was that analgesic efficacy would be associated with just one of these subtypes and adverse effects with others. This has not quite been the case; many of the drugs acting on these receptor subtypes lack the full analgesic efficacy of morphine (Table 7-3).

---

[1]Schedule I drugs may only be used for research.

[2]Unfortunately there are no accurate records.
[3]Sigmund Freud tried to treat morphine addiction with cocaine but concluded that it was "like trying to cast out the Devil with Beelzebub."

TABLE 7-3 Opioid Receptors: Ligands, Locations, and Functions

IUPHAR NOMENCLATURE	"TRADITIONAL" NOMENCLATURE	ENDOGENOUS LIGANDS	CNS LOCATIONS	FUNCTIONS
MOP	Mu, μ (μ_1, μ_2, μ_3)	β-Endorphin Enkephalin Endomorphin-1 Endomorphin-2	Cerebral cortex Thalamus Periaqueductal gray (Analgesia) Spinal cord	μ_1 Supraspinal analgesia Physical dependence μ_2 Respiratory depression Miosis **Euphoria** ↓ GI motility Physical dependence
DOP	Delta, δ (δ_1, δ_2)	Enkephalins β-Endorphin	Pontine nuclei Amygdala Olfactory bulbs Deep cortex	Analgesia Antidepressant Physical dependence
KOP	Kappa, κ (κ, κ_2, κ_3)	Dynorphin A Dynorphin B α-Neoendorphin	Hypothalamus (Reward) Periaqueductal gray Spinal cord	Spinal analgesia Sedation Miosis ↓ Antidiuretic hormone release
NOP	Nociceptin (ORL_1)	Nociceptin/ Orphanin FQ	Cortex Amygdala Hippocampus Hypothalamus Spinal cord	Anxiolytic Antidepressant Decreased appetite Tolerance to μ agonists

© Delmar/Cengage Learning

What makes the situation more complicated is that not all drugs that bind to opioid receptors are full agonists that only activate receptors and are always analgesic (Table 7-4). These include morphine, methadone, oxycodone (Percocet, Oxycontin), and codeine. Other drugs are pure antagonists, which always block these receptors and are used as antidotes for opioid overdoses. These include naloxone (Narcan) and naltrexone (ReVia).

Complicating the issue is a group of drugs known as agonist-antagonists or mixed agonists. These drugs, which include nalbuphine (Nubain) and butorphanol (Stadol), are moderately effective analgesics when given alone because they are KOP receptor agonists (Table 7-4). However—and here is where it gets complicated—when given to an opioid dependent patient, these drugs can precipitate withdrawal, because they are MOP receptor antagonists as well. Clinically, mixed agonists should never be used to wean a patient off morphine or any other full agonist.

The last class of opioid drugs is the partial agonists such as buprenorphine (Buprenex, Subutex, Suboxone). A partial agonist combines with a receptor but produces weaker effects than those of the full agonist. As a partial MOP receptor agonist, buprenorphine decreases cravings for other opioids, prevents opioid withdrawal, and is less sedating than full MOP-opioid agonists. Buprenorphine also has a "ceiling effect." That is, high doses of the drug do not produce the same euphoric effects as those of pure MOP agonists and it also has a lower abuse potential. Buprenorphine is often used to prevent relapse in opioid addicted patients (Srivastava & Kahan, 2006). It has been speculated that buprenorphine's agonist effect at the NOP receptor may confer to the drug mild antidepressant properties.

A logical question to ask here is, Why do humans have receptors for chemicals found in plants that grow almost exclusively in Middle East countries (such as Afghanistan)? Reasoning that these receptors must exist for endogenous agonists fulfilling a physiological function, led researchers in the 1970s to discover a series of brain peptides that had morphine-like activity. Since then several others have been identified (Corbett et al., 2006). Table 7-3 summarizes the

TABLE 7-4 Opioid Receptor Agonists and Antagonists

	FULL AGONIST	PARTIAL AGONIST	ANTAGONIST
MOP (Mu)	Morphine Methadone Oxycodone Codeine	Buprenorphine	Naloxone Naltrexone Nalbuphine Butorphanol
KOP (Kappa)	Nalbuphine Butorphanol	THC(??)	Buprenorphine
NOP (Nociceptin)		Buprenorphine	–

© Delmar/Cengage Learning

locations in the central nervous system of both opioid receptors and the endogenous opioids and relates them, as much as possible, to physiological functions and pharmacological activity.

Pharmacology and Pharmacotherapy

Table 7-5 shows the wide range of action that opioids have on structures throughout the body. These drugs act not only in the brain and spinal cord to decrease pain perception and reaction to pain (anxiety, suffering); they also act on numerous other tissues, making this class of drugs quite useful, but with numerous adverse effects, too.

ANXIOLYTIC–SEDATIVE– HYPNOTICS

The anxiolytic–sedative–hypnotics produce dose-related central nervous system depression and are used clinically to reduce anxiety and to facilitate and maintain sleep. Excessive doses of many drugs in this class have the potential to depress respiration and cause death. Throughout history people have used chemicals to relax and to sleep, yet, few chemicals were effective and fewer still were both safe and effective. Prior to the 1900s only a handful of sedatives were in clinical use. These included bromide, chloral hydrate, and paraldehyde. The first barbiturate, phenobarbital, was introduced in 1912, followed by many others in the next few decades. None of these drugs were effective anxiolytics, or at least none were effective at reducing anxiety while the patient was awake. In other words, the anxiolytic and hypnotic doses could not be teased apart.

That all changed in 1961 with the introduction of chlordiazepoxide (Librium) followed a year later by diazepam (Valium), a drug 3 to 10 times as potent and with a wider range of activity. For the first time, daytime anxiety could be controlled with minimal sedation. Today benzodiazepines are used for anxiety (e.g., lorazepam—Ativan), insomnia (triazolam—Halcion), epilepsy (diazepam—Valium), muscle relaxation (diazepam—Valium), and induction of anesthesia (midazolam—Versed). Almost all benzodiazepines, at appropriate doses, can be used for all of these purposes. Because of their safety—it is almost impossible to take a lethal dose of a benzodiazepine in the absence of other drugs—benzodiazepines have more or less become the de facto standard drugs of choice for insomnia and anxiety.

In the last decade and a half, a new group of drugs (the "Z" hypnotics), including zolpidem (Ambien), zapelon (Sonata), and eszopiclone (Lunesta) have been introduced into clinical practice. While structurally distinct from the benzodiazepines, these drugs bind to a particular benzodiazepine receptor subtype and are selective for treating insomnia. These drugs do not reduce anxiety, relax aching muscles, or stop seizures.

Mechanism of Action

The action of the benzodiazepines and the barbiturates via the $GABA_A$ receptor in the brain, discussed in detail in Chapter 6, is worth a brief review. The $GABA_A$ receptor consists of five meticulously arranged peptide subunits embedded in the neuronal membrane. The five subunits (out of a potential 16 subunits) can combine in different ways to form $GABA_A$ receptors, and *how* they combine determines the receptor's agonist affinity, chance of opening a chloride channel, conductance, and other properties (Barnard et al., 1998; Olsen & Sieghart, 2008). At the junction of these subunits are secondary or allosteric binding sites to which certain drugs can bind and modulate the primary binding site for GABA, affecting both the frequency and duration of Cl^- channel openings. One such allosteric site on the $GABA_A$ receptor complex binds benzodiazepines (Lydiard, 2003). Other allosteric modulators include barbiturates and ethanol. When bound to the allosteric site sites, these drugs have anxiolytic, anticonvulsant, amnestic, sedative, hypnotic, euphoric, and muscle-relaxing actions.

Pharmacology and Pharmacotherapy

Barbiturates are infrequently used in clinical practice except for epilepsy (phenobarbital) and for the induction of anesthesia (thiopental). Unlike the benzodiazepines, these drugs depress all electrically excitable tissue, affecting not only nervous tissue (i.e., the brain), but they also depress cardiac and respiratory muscles at high doses, making them potentially lethal drugs. In the 1950s and 1960s death in barbiturate abusers was much higher than with any other abused drugs. "Drug automatism" (i.e., patient takes the drug, gets groggy and confused, and takes additional doses) with barbiturates was all too common. Moreover, chronic use of barbiturates induces ("soups up") liver enzymes, altering the metabolism of other drugs and increases the risk of adverse drug reactions.

TABLE 7-5 Opioid Actions on Organ Systems

ORGAN SYSTEM/TISSUE	ACTIONS
Central Nervous System	
Cortex	• Decreased pain perception • Altered reaction to pain • Patient can tolerate more pain • **Euphoria** or dysphoria • Sedation/hypnosis
Medulla	• Thermoregulation • Respiratory depression • Reduces coughing • Causes nausea and vomiting • Vasomotor depression
Spinal cord	• Stimulates most reflexes and spinal functions • Depresses reflexes related to pain
Nucleus of the occulomotor nerve	• Pinpoint pupils
Vagus nerve	• Bradycardia • Increased gastrointestinal tone
Gastrointestinal Tract	• Constipative and spasmogenic • Decreases propulsive contractions and increases segmental contractions • Decreases defecation reflex—decreases tone of pyloric and anal sphincters
Other Smooth Muscle	• Bronchiolar constriction (at high doses) • Bile duct (increased biliary pressure) • Uterus (labor prolonged) • Ureters (difficulty urinating)
Histamine Release	• Postural hypotension • Cutaneous flushing and itching

© Delmar/Cengage Learning

Low margins of safety, high probability of drug interactions, and frequent abuse facilitated the rapid switch from barbiturates to benzodiazepines almost immediately after these were introduced into clinical practice.

Benzodiazepines are far more selective than older drugs. For most patients, low doses of these drugs can adequately control anxiety without causing sedation. Although they too are CNS depressants, benzodiazepines do not affect cardiac or respiratory muscle, nor do they alter liver enzymes to affect drug metabolism. Thus, they have fewer adverse effects, are safer, and are less likely to interfere with the action of other drugs.

There are, however, issues that must be considered when benzodiazepines are used. First, when used for sleep, their effects may persist into daytime hours, potentially interfering with daily functions, especially in elderly patients. Second,

benzodiazepines can cause anterograde amnesia (i.e., new events are not transferred to long-term memory after taking the drug), particularly with high doses or when combined with alcohol. The prototype scoundrel for this issue is flunitrazepam (Rohypnol), an exquisitely potent benzodiazepine (not approved for clinical use in the United States). The drug can profoundly affect the memory of the "user" for several hours after consumption. Because of its high potency, it can be combined with alcoholic beverages without altering the taste. For this reason, as we previously noted in Chapter 6, Rohypnol is commonly referred to as the "date-rape" drug.

An additional advantage of benzodiazepines over older drugs is the availability of an antidote for severe overdose. Just as naloxone (Narcan) can be used to reverse the effects of opioids, flumazenil (Romazicon) can reverse the effects of benzodiazepines. Flumazenil is an antagonist at the allosteric binding site for benzodiazepines on the GABA$_A$ receptor complex.

The non-benzodiazepine benzodiazepine-receptor agonists (zolpidem, zapelon, and eszopiclone) are even more selective than the benzodiazepines, affecting only one function, sleep. However, in recent years several reports of rare (less than 1:1000 patients) unusual nighttime behaviors in patients taking zolpidem have been reported. These include sleepwalking (somnambulism), sleep-driving, sleep-eating, and rare reports of hallucinations. As yet, there are no scientific explanations for these behaviors.

PSYCHOSTIMULANTS

Amphetamine was first synthesized in Germany in 1887. In 1919, Japanese scientists discovered that by slightly modifying the drug with the strategic addition of a methyl group they had developed a more potent form of the drug, methamphetamine, which could be injected or taken orally. In the 1920s, scientists found that amphetamine constricted blood vessels and dilated bronchial passages and reduced drowsiness by stimulating the central nervous system. By the 1930s, Benzedrine was marketed over-the-counter in the United States to treat nasal congestion. Two commonly reported effects of the drug when taken orally were "a sense of well-being and a feeling of exhilaration" and "lessened fatigue in reaction to work." During World War II, American and British pilots were routinely issued amphetamines to combat fatigue and heighten endurance. (Ironically, Germany and Japan developed drugs that were used by Allied forces.)

It did not take long for the amphetamines to become abused substances. Amphetamines are known on the street as speed, zip, dexies, bennies, bumblebees, cross tops, jellybeans, uppers, and crank. By the 1950s, tablets of methamphetamine (Methedrine) and dextroamphetamine (Dexedrine) were legally manufactured and became available to the public. Truck drivers, athletes, and executives (ab)used them and students popped them to cram for exams. Amphetamines were also used, mostly by women, as weight-control pills. These drugs became ingrained in the society of the 1960s. This all changed in 1971, when the United States passed the Controlled Substances Act and the amphetamines were classified as Schedule II drugs.

Today, the two primary accepted clinical uses of amphetamines are to treat narcolepsy and ADHD. Although it seems counterintuitive, psychostimulants can improve impulse control and concentration, decrease sensory overstimulation and irritability, and appear to reduce anxiety, as well (see Chapter 5).

Methylphenidate (Ritalin), first synthesized in 1944, did not begin clinical trials for another decade. By 1957 it was marketed to treat chronic fatigue, depression, and narcolepsy, and to reverse sedation caused by other drugs, including barbiturates. In the late 1950s and early 1960s, it was evaluated as a possible treatment of ADHD, then called "hyperkinetic syndrome." Today, it is the primary drug used to treat ADHD and is sold in immediate-release and extended- or sustained-release (Ritalin SR, Ritalin LA, Metadate ER, Metadate CD, Methylin ER, and Concerta) preparations. Because of its abuse potential, methylphenidate (Vitamin R, Rit, Kibbles and Bits, Pineapple, and West Coast) is a DEA Schedule II drug.

Mechanism of Action

Amphetamine produces multiple dose-dependent actions on neurons that release norepinephrine (NE—noradrenergic, Figure 7-1) and dopamine (DA—dopaminergic). At low, ADHD-therapeutic doses, amphetamine facilitates the release of NE and DA from presynaptic neurons throughout the nervous system. With higher (toxic) doses, it also blocks the reuptake of neuronally released NE (and DA), elevating synaptic levels of the NT still further. At very high (lethal) doses, amphetamine also inhibits intraneuronal metabolism of NE, so that when an action potential arrives at the axon terminal, more NT is released per action potential. The overall effect of amphetamine is to raise neuronal levels of both NE and DA (and, perhaps, 5-HT), by one or more mechanisms of action.

Methylphenidate (Ritalin) is more selective than amphetamine. Methylphenidate (actually d,l-threo-methylphenidate, MPH) acts primarily by inhibiting presynaptic DA reuptake, and much less so on NE reuptake (Findling, 2008; Patrick et al., 2005).

Amphetamine and amphetamine-like drugs are nonselective in that they act in the brain and in the periphery to raise neurotransmitter (NT) levels, causing many adverse effects (Table 7-6). Amphetamine is manufactured as a racemic mixture of two isomers (chemically identical mirror images), dextro-amphetamine (d-) and levo-amphetamine (l-).

Whereas dextroamphetamine acts more on the brain, levoamphetamine acts more on the cardiovascular system. From a clinical perspective, the desirable effects (improved attentiveness and focus) of amphetamine are conferred to the d-isomer, and the adverse effects (tachycardia, hypertension) to the l-isomer. Currently, l-amphetamine is only available in

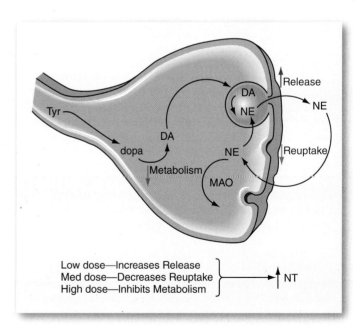

FIGURE 7-1 Synthesis, release, reuptake, and metabolism of norepinephrine in neurons. As the dose of amphetamines is increased, the drug first increases release of NE, then blocks reuptake, and finally inhibits its metabolism by the enzyme monoamine oxidase (MAO). Similar actions occur in dopaminergic neurons in brain.

TABLE 7-6 Psychostimulant Drug Actions

THERAPEUTIC - DESIRED	IMMEDIATE TOXICITY	LONG-TERM ISSUES
• Appetite suppression • Wakefulness • Heightened alertness • Euphoria	• Impairment of voluntary movement • Headache • Irregular or rapid heartbeat • Nausea and vomiting • Skin rash • Exhilaration and excitation • Agitation • Muscle twitching • Dilation of pupils • Confusion • Hallucinations and paranoia • Flushing • Increased blood pressure and heart rate • Dry mouth • Vomiting • Fever and sweating • Delirium • Seizures, followed by coma • Anxiety and restlessness • Excessive repetition of movements and meaningless tasks • Formication—the sensation of bugs or worms crawling under the skin	• Pronounced fatigue • Malnutrition • Neglected hygiene • Hair loss • Involuntary movement disorders • Sexual dysfunction • Cerebrovascular damage • Weight loss (possibly substantial) • Nose bleed from intranasal ingestion • Muscle cramping from dehydration and depleted electrolytes • Dermatological conditions • Constipation from dehydration and lack of dietary fiber

mixed amphetamine salt preparations such as Adderall and Adderall XR, whereas d-amphetamine is available in these preparations and as a free-standing drug for ADHD and narcolepsy (Dexedrine and DextoStat).

As with amphetamine, methylphenidate (MPH) is synthesized as a racemic mixture of d- and l-isomers and, until quite recently, this has been the only form available. A 2008 review of the relevant literature by Markowitz and Patrick (2008) suggests that all the pharmacological activity resides with the d-isomer. If anything, the data also suggests that the l-isomer may counter the beneficial neurophysiological action of d-MPH. As such, availability of a drug preparation containing only d-MPH should have marked clinical advantages over existing drugs (McGough, Pataki, & Suddath, 2005). Focalin and Focalin XR are two forms of dexmethylphenidate used to treat ADHD.

Pharmacology and Pharmacotherapy

Psychostimulants raise both central and peripheral levels of DA and NE. The therapeutic effects on behavior are mediated by these neurotransmitters in the brain whereas the adverse effects are due to both central (anxiety, restlessness, hallucinations, paranoia, seizures) and peripheral (rapid heartbeat, elevated blood pressure, headache, flushing) effects (Table 7-6). Since DA has little neurotransmitter action outside of the brain, most peripheral adverse effects of these drugs are due to the action of NE. In addition to the acute adverse effects, chronic use/abuse of the psychostimulants can lead to

additional health problems including pronounced fatigue, malnutrition, sexual dysfunction, weight loss, etc. (Table 7-6).

Although the stimulants had a long clinical history dating back to the late 1800s, they had only two acceptable clinical uses: to combat sleepiness (central action) and to dilate bronchioles in asthmatic patients (peripheral action). Certainly no one would dream of giving an amphetamine to children, especially hyperactive children, would they? That is, until Charles Bradley, the medical director of the Emma Pendleton Bradley Home, decided to try it. His paper (1937), published without much fanfare, might have revolutionized the treatment of hyperactive children had more clinicians read it and at least attempted to replicate his findings. In what is now considered a seminal study, Bradley reported that 14 of 30 children with behavior problems showed a "spectacular change in behavior . . . remarkably improved school performance" during one week of treatment with Benzedrine. However, it took another quarter century before the psychostimulants became the mainstay therapy for ADHD. Why did it take so long to catch on? It was simply poor timing on Bradley's part; his observations and paper came before the age of biological psychiatry was accepted as reality. At the time of his report, psychological intervention, not drugs, was the only accepted treatment for childhood behavioral disorders.

The psychostimulants (Table 7-7) are available in immediate-release/rapid-onset/short-duration formulations (2 to 6 hours) and as extended-or slow-release preparations (8 to 12 hours). Although both forms of amphetamines and

TABLE 7-7 Psychostimulant Preparations

	AMPHETAMINE/ DEXTROAMPHETAMINE	METHYLPHENIDATE/ DEXMETHYLPHENIDATE
Immediate Release	Adderall	Ritalin
	Dexedrine	Methylin
	Dextrostat	Focalin
	Desoxyn (Methamphetamine)	
Extended Release	Adderall XR	Ritalin SR
	Dexedrine SR	Ritalin LA
	Dexedrine Spansule	Metadate ER
	Vynase (Lisdexamfetamine)	Metadate CD
		Methylin ER
		Concerta
		Focalin XR
		Daytrana (Transdermal patch)

© Delmar/Cengage Learning

methylphenidate are equally effective in managing ADHD, the slow-release preparations offer a number of advantages in day-to-day management of this disorder. Immediate-release preparations kick in right away but must be given multiple times throughout the day to be effective.

In the United States, ADHD is diagnosed in an estimated 8% of school children ages 6 to 17, of whom almost 60% are treated with medication (Pastor, 2008). With immediate-onset, short-acting drugs, schools have the responsibility of monitoring drug administration during the day. The use of extended-release preparations, if nothing else, removes this undue burden on the schools. Moreover, abuse of psychostimulants in high schools may be reduced with greater parental control over distribution and administration.

ADHD does not vanish along with acne at the end of adolescence; it continues into adulthood for many people. Kessler and his colleagues (2006) estimate the prevalence of ADHD is 4.4% in adults. Moreover, its prevalence into adulthood is directly proportional to the severity of ADHD in childhood. Kessler did not observe ADHD in people who did not experience it growing up. The prevalence of ADHD (as determined by trained clinical interviewers) was 7% in people with subthreshold childhood symptoms and was up to about 37% in those who had full childhood criteria but denied having current symptoms of ADHD. The reason this data is included in this chapter, and not in Chapter 5, is because the abuse of the psychostimulants is most likely to occur in college-age adults, for whom there is not adult supervision of dosing and who may be under great stress, particularly around the time of finals.

SELECTIVE ABUSE

Drug addicts are generally selective in the drugs they tend to abuse. They abuse specific drugs for specific reasons and generally do not interchange drugs haphazardly when the desired drug is not available. Each of these drugs produces a specific euphoria and each is used for different reasons. For example, the singing legend Elvis Presley infamously used an array of downers. His autopsy results yielded as many as 13 different drugs in his bloodstream at the time of his death.[4]

OPIOIDS

When life is not going well, opioids and alcohol tend to be the abused drugs of choice. Under the influence of opioids users become indifferent to their surroundings. By taking some oxycodone (Oxycontin, Percocet) or heroin, one might feel that life's problems seem to vanish, at least for a few hours. The trouble with this approach, however, is that when the drug wears off, the problems still exist. So the choice is to take more drugs, and the cycle continues.

ALCOHOL AND ANXIOLYTIC– SEDATIVE–HYPNOTICS

Why is alcohol a drug that is commonly abused by artists, musicians, and writers? Because alcohol produces something known as "disinhibition euphoria." When someone is looking for the right metaphor, the perfect note, or flawless brushstroke and it doesn't pop into the conscious mind because it is hopelessly "inhibited," a little nip of rum just may help free things up. Sometimes alcohol is used to deal with unexpressed anger, or feelings of insecurity or awkwardness. When alcohol's disinhibition euphoria kicks in, people "feel better" and are less inhibited about themselves or their behavior. Those

---

[4]When Elvis "The King" Presley (1935–1977) died of a cardiac arrhythmia in his modest home, Graceland, an autopsy showed the following drugs coursing through his bloodstream: morphine, meperidine, chlorpheniramine, ethchlorvynol, diazepam, ethinamate, methaqualone, an unknown barbiturate, and possibly amobarbital, pentobarbital, carbromal, amitriptyline, and nortriptyline. Not an upper or a street drug among them.

who can't risk smelling of alcohol might resort to taking a pill, and not just any pill; it should be a benzodiazepine because it has similar effects to alcohol but no odor.

PSYCHOSTIMULANTS

The two most common psychostimulants used in the United States do not require prescriptions and are a common part of the American morning schedule. The first is caffeine, found in coffee, tea, or cola beverages and the second is nicotine, found in tobacco products. These stimulants are consumed to increase alertness and to combat tedium and monotony. While caffeine is still a widely accepted part of American life and a symbol of better living through nature's chemistry, nicotine has not fared so well in recent years. The problem is not so much the nicotine itself but the delivery vehicle for the drug, cigarettes. These white cylinders filled with tightly packed tobacco leaves produce cancer-inducing byproducts when burned. These byproducts are inhaled as part of the process of delivering nicotine to the lungs where it is absorbed and then, at lightning speed, delivered to the brain.

But this section is not about nicotine or caffeine-like stimulants. It's about drugs—amphetamine, methamphetamine, and cocaine—that markedly elevate DA levels in the brain. Elevating DA in the right areas (nucleus accumbens and ventral tegmentum, for example) is quite pleasurable and rewarding, and once again, as B. F. Skinner so adroitly proved, "behavior (smoking methamphetamine) followed by a reinforcing stimulus (euphoria comparable to whole body orgasm) results in an increased probability of that behavior occurring in the future (addiction)." These stimulants are among the most effective positive reinforcers known to man and are among the most addictive drugs. (Ab)users frequently take them to produce a sense of exhilaration, improve self-esteem, expand mental and physical performance, increase activity, diminish hunger, stay awake longer, study harder, enhance sexual performance, and feel high.

ISSUES OF COMORBIDITY

Comorbidity between mental illness (depression, bipolar disorder, anxiety) and substance abuse disorders is not infrequent (Cerda, Sagdeo, & Galea, 2008; Quello, Brady, & Sonne, 2005). A question often asked is which issue came first—the mental health problem or the substance abuse. One side argues—quite logically—that drugs are abused to self-medicate mental distress. Most problems temporarily vanish if enough opioid is taken. Alcohol helps writer's block, and amphetamines provide the stimulation to cram for an exam for two days continuously and remember everything. However, maybe this sequence is backwards and the use of these powerfully potent chemicals changes brain neurochemistry such that the user gets anxious, depressed, manic, or psychotic.

Several studies have examined this enigma. The problem is that trying to answer the question with an either-or scenario is a straw man argument, in that it assumes only two possible answers: the chicken (mental illness) is first or the egg (substance abuse) is first. This response ignores the more complex answer that they are related but can occur independently. Now—and this may be more challenging—think of the brain

as a hen house filled with many chickens and many eggs. Because the conditions are ideally suited for both laying and hatching to occur, chickens can lay eggs and eggs can hatch chickens.

A person's genetic makeup at conception combined with environmental conditions during development (gestation through adulthood) create a self-contained biopsychological crucible where all the ingredients mix and swirl, resulting in the *perfect storm*[5] for either mental illness or substance abuse or both to occur. A systematic review (Cerda et al., 2008) of dozens of peer-reviewed articles has shown significant comorbidities among these populations but no cause-and-effect relationship in the direction of change (i.e., does one always come first?). Comorbidity between mental health issues and substance use disorders may exist because of overlapping neurobiological pathways, common underlying genetic factors, and diagnostic confounding (Quello et al., 2005). Most people develop normally with neither substance abuse nor mental health problems.

THE SUBSTRATE OF ADDICTION

The last few sections of this chapter cover the neuroanatomical sites for three classes of prescription psychoactive drugs with abuse potential: opioids used to treat pain anxiolytic-sedative-hypnotics to lessen anxiety and reduce insomnia and psychostimulants to improve ADHD and control narcolepsy.

This leads to an important question. Are the same brain sites and the same neurotransmitters also responsible for the abuse potential of these drugs? Stated another way, is addiction to opioids of necessity mediated by changes in endogenous opioid pathways, addiction to benzodiazepines by the alterations in the $GABA_A$ receptor complex, and addiction to cocaine and amphetamines via modified DA pathways? Or, could there be a common neurochemical thread running through all forms of addiction, regardless of reinforcer, whether it be morphine, diazepam, cocaine, nicotine, marijuana, gambling, sex, or food. If there is a universal substrate for addiction and addictive behaviors, what is it, and does it imply that science could develop a universal antidote or treatment for all addiction?

The single neurotransmitter that seems to fit the bill is dopamine, and the principal area of the brain affected would be the mesolimbic dopamine pathway traversing from the ventral tegmental area (VTA) in the midbrain to the nucleus accumbens (NA) in the limbic system and to the prefrontal cortex in the cerebrum (Figure 7-2). More than 20 years of research support this hypothesis (Di Chiara, 1999; Robinson & Berridge, 1993). Most abused substances, including alcohol and nicotine, directly or indirectly elevate dopamine activity in this pathway (Esch & Stefano, 2004). The positively reinforcing effects (i.e., euphoria) of dopamine, would lead to repetition of whatever behavior

---

[5]Based on the title of the book by Sebastian Junger. The phrase *perfect storm* has gained popularity and grown to mean any event where a combination of circumstances will aggravate a situation drastically. Incidentally, the phrase was awarded the top prize by Lake Superior State University in its 2007 list of words that deserve to be banned for overuse.

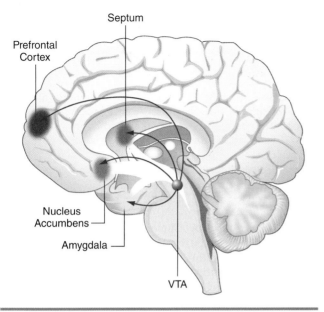

FIGURE 7-2 Dopamine pathways of rewards beginning at the ventral Tegmental area (VTA) to the amygdala, nucleus accumbens, septum, and prefrontal cortex.

that had led to its elevation, hence continued or habitual use of drug.

However, there is accumulating evidence that another neurotransmitter, glutamate (GLU), may also be involved in addiction (Gass & Olive, 2008; Uys & LaLumiere, 2008). This is where Homer, a family of proteins, gets involved (Szumlinski, Ary, & Lominac, 2008). Homer proteins play a role in regulating the functional architecture of GLU synapses, perhaps as part of the molecular scaffolding in the communication between GLU receptor actions and calcium-related cellular events (Szumlinski et al., 2008).

Before discussing the role of Homer proteins in addiction, it is important to return to the neurotransmitter GLU and its potentially overarching role as a—or the—chemical substrate for addiction. Perhaps it took so long to elucidate the functional significance of GLU in addiction because GLU is a ubiquitous molecule in the brain. It is believed to mediate as much as 70% of all synaptic neurotransmission in the CNS. Moreover, it is released not only by neurons but by glial cells (astrocytes) as well. Furthermore, whereas the concentration of most NTs in the brain is in the nano- to micromolar range, GLU concentration in some cells may be in the millimolar range (i.e., thousands to millions of times greater than other NTs). Trying to identify specific roles for GLU is not just trying to find the needle in a haystack—it is more like trying to find one particular bit of hay in all the haystacks on a farm. In recent years the availability of sophisticated analytical tools, better understanding of GLU receptor subtypes, and the synthesis of highly selective ligands has increased the understanding of this transmitter's role in learning and memory (see Chapter 5) and now, in addiction.

One reason that dopamine was hypothesized as a potential substrate for addiction is that its neuroanatomical distribution is in precisely the regions of the brain that such a chemical is expected to be found—that is, in the reward circuitry (Figure 7-2). However, DA is not there in isolation, independent of other neurotransmitters. In fact, as shown in Table 7-8, each stop along the mesolimbic DA pathway seems to crisscross with a GLU pathway (Gass & Olive, 2008). In their review of the salient literature, Gass and Olive (2008) point out that many of the acute (therapeutic) and chronic (dependence, tolerance, and addiction) effects of opioids, cocaine, amphetamine, nicotine, cannabinoids (marijuana, THC), and alcohol may be at least partially mediated by GLU. Moreover, in the hippocampus, GLU is a key player in

TABLE 7-8 Glutamate (GLU) input to the Mesolimbic DA "Reward Circuit"

MESOLIMBIC DA "REWARD CIRCUIT" NEUROANATOMICAL FOCI	RECEIVES GLU INPUT FROM . . .
Ventral Tegmental Area	Pedunculopontine tegmentum Lateral dorsal tegmentum Amygdala Frontal cortex
Nucleus Accumbens	Frontal cortex Hippocampus Thalamus Amygdala
Amygdala	Hippocampus Frontal cortex
Frontal Cortex	Hippocampus Thalamus Amygdala

learning, memory, and synaptic plasticity (see Chapter 1)—and what are drug dependence and tolerance if not exemplars of drug-induced plasticity.

GLU is also a target in addiction research because several glutamatergic drugs have been found to decrease drug craving, diminish their use, and ease the symptoms of withdrawal in humans or in animal models for these conditions (Gass & Olive, 2008). Examples of glutamatergic drugs include acamprosate, N-acetyl-cysteine, modafinil, topiramate, lamotrigine, and memantine. Importantly, several of these drugs have proved beneficial with more than one class of abused compounds—as shown in Table 7-9—suggesting a common molecular agent for addiction.

What is Homer's role in addiction, particularly in regard to the neurotransmitter glutamate? It has been speculated that the repetitive and continuous use of abused substances usurps molecular mechanisms of synaptic plasticity within relevant areas of the brain (Robinson & Kolb, 2004). In the prefrontal cortex and in the nucleus accumbens, at dendritic spines, where postsynaptic contact for over 90% of excitatory synapses occur, changes in the neuronal morphology has been reported when exposed to drugs of abuse. These dendritic spines are rich in neurotransmitter receptors and contain the obligatory intraneuronal infrastructure required to make them functionally relevant. Cocaine, amphetamine, morphine, nicotine, and alcohol have all been shown to alter spine density and branching in key brain regions involved in addiction.

Critical molecules for regulating dendritic morphology are Homers. Szumlinski and colleagues (Szumlinski, Kalivas, & Worley, 2006) theorize that Homer proteins, critical in regulating synaptic architecture of glutamatergic neurons, also regulate addiction vulnerability by causing morphological changes. Szumlinski reports in her paper that changes in various Homer proteins in one or more regions of the brain occur after cocaine, alcohol, methamphetamine, nicotine, LSD, PCP, and morphine administration.

So, is this the purported Philosopher's Stone[6] of addiction, the mysterious fundamental molecule underlying all

addiction? Probably not, but perhaps it is one step closer in understanding the neurochemistry of addiction.

ABSTINENCE INITIATION

If there is a single neurochemical responsible for all addiction, its identity is as yet unknown. If such a molecule exists it might be possible to treat all addiction with just one drug. In addition to a wide range of behavioral approaches, several drugs are in use today to facilitate abstinence initiation in drug addicts or to help them with relapse prevention. Table 7-10 summarizes the drugs currently in use or under investigation for opioid, stimulant, nicotine, and alcohol use disorders.

The Food and Drug Administration (FDA) has approved one or more drugs to treat substance abuse disorders, particularly for opioids, nicotine, and alcohol. Numerous tactics have been employed to this end. These include drugs that work by the identical mechanism used by the abused drugs but are longer acting (e.g., methadone), drugs that are partial agonists (e.g., buprenorphine), and drugs that are receptor antagonists (e.g., naltrexone) at the receptor for the abused drug. However, there are at least two drugs (naltrexone and disulfiram) used to treat addiction whose mechanism of action are making us rethink our understanding of the addictive process.

OPIOIDS

In the Woody Allen movie *Annie Hall*, a character recalling his life uttered the sardonically humorous line, "I used to be a heroin addict. Now I'm a methadone addict." Methadone maintenance, available since the 1960s, is a rational and sensible form of addiction therapy based on the idea that addicts with many years of illegal drug use cannot suddenly stop using drugs altogether and immediately re-enter society and become productive citizens. Providing drug addicts with a legal source of drug in a safe and healthy medical environment has been shown to reduce illicit opioid use; diminish the risk of contracting and transmitting HIV, tuberculosis, and hepatitis; and eliminate the need to engage illegal activities to fund the behavior (Krambeer, von McKnelly, Gabrielli, & Penick, 2001). While in treatment, users can engage in reinforceable, socially accepted behaviors (e.g., working for a salary), so that the unacceptable behavior (e.g., intravenous heroin

---

[6]"A conjectural and, in fact, imaginary substance capable of transmuting base metals into gold. Its discovery and preparation was the fruitless task of alchemists from early China and India, by way of medieval Arabs, down to various Faust-like figures of the Renaissance such as Paracelsus. It was a solid variant of the liquid elixir of life. The alchemists' pursuit of it led to the acquisition of much genuine chemical knowledge and, indeed, to the foundation of chemistry as a science." (The Rt. Hon. Lord Quinton, *The Oxford Companion to Philosophy*, 2005).

TABLE 7-9 Glutamate and Drug Addiction

GLUTAMATERIGIC DRUG	DRUG ADDICTION (INCLUDES DECREASED CRAVING, USE, AND SEVERITY OF WITHDRAWAL)
Acamprosate (Campral)	Alcohol, cocaine, opioids
N-acetyl-cysteine	Cocaine
Modafinil (Provigil)	Cocaine
Topiramate (Topamax)	Opioids, benzodiazepines, cocaine, nicotine, alcohol
Lamotrigine (Lamictal)	Cocaine, alcohol, inhalants
Memantine (Namenda)	Alcohol, opioids

TABLE 7-10 Summary of Drugs Used to Treat Drug Addiction

DRUG	MECHANISM OF ACTION	FDA APPROVAL
Opioids		
Methadone	Partial opioid receptor agonist	1960s
Buprenorphine (Subutex, Suboxone)	Partial opioid receptor agonist	2002
Naltrexone (ReVia)	Opioid receptor antagonist	1984
Stimulants		
Disulfiram (Antabuse)	Blocks metabolism of dopamine (and ethanol)	
Aripiprazole (Abilify)	Partial DA receptor agonist	
Modafinil (Provigil)	GLU agonist (also α_1 agonist and NE reuptake blocker)	
Memantine (Namenda)	GLU (NMDA) receptor antagonist	None approved
Lamotrigine (Lamictal)	Decreases presynaptic release of GLU	
Topiramate (Topamax)	Blocks GLU (AMPA and kainate) receptors. Enhanced GABAA activity	
Gabapentin (Neurontin)	Decreases breakdown of GABA	
Tiagabine (Gabitril)	Blocks GABA reuptake	
Nicotine		
Nicotine	Replacement therapy	
Bupropion (Zyban)	Likely mediated by NE and/or DA mechanisms	1997
Varenicline (Chantix)	High affinity, partial agonist at the $\alpha_4\beta_2$ nicotinic acetylcholine receptor	2006
Naltrexone (ReVia)	Opioid receptor antagonist. Basis for reducing nicotine consumption is unknown.	In clinical trials
Alcohol		
Naltrexone (ReVia)	Opioid receptor antagonist. Basis for reducing alcohol consumption is unknown.	1995
Acamprosate (Campral)	GLU (NMDA) receptor antagonist, activation of GABA$_A$ receptors	2004
Disulfiram (Antabuse)	Blocks metabolism of ethanol (and dopamine)	1983

use) is extinguished (Skinner, 1938). Methadone maintenance therapy provides the time for this transition to occur. In some ways the Woody Allen joke is correct: the addiction is switched from an illegal drug to a legal drug. But once that is attained, it should be easier for clinicians to deal with the behavior that maintains the substance abuse disorder.

Buprenorphine (Subutex, Suboxone) is an example of a drug that takes another approach to treating the opioid-addicted patient. This drug is a partial MOP-opioid receptor agonist. Its maximal effects are less than those of full agonists such as heroin and morphine. At low doses, buprenorphine has sufficient MOP-opioid agonist activity to enable opioid-addicted individuals to discontinue use of full opioid agonists (morphine, oxycodone, heroin) without experiencing withdrawal symptoms but at higher doses the drug reaches a "ceiling effect," and the user cannot attain the level of euphoria (i.e., high) of a full agonist. Thus, buprenorphine carries a lower risk of abuse, dependence, and side effects compared to full opioid agonists. It has been speculated that the antagonist action of buprenorphine at DOP receptors may explain why tolerance to the drug does not develop. Buprenorphine is used clinically to both facilitate abstinence and to prevent relapse.

In addition, studies as early as 1995 indicate that buprenorphine may also be effective in treating mild depression (Bodkin, Zornberg, Lukas, & Cole, 1995). Recent anecdotal evidence suggests that it has a rapid onset of action (perhaps hours) and now the NIH is actively enrolling patients to test buprenorphine's effectiveness in acutely suicidal patients. (*A Double-Blind Study of Buprenorphine Treatment of Acute Suicidality—ClinicalTrials.gov.*). This action, interestingly, may be mediated by buprenorphine at the NOP (nociceptin) receptor (McCann, 2008).

Naltrexone (ReVia) is an orally effective pure opioid receptor antagonist. Since it was approved in 1984 to treat opioid addiction, it has been an invaluable medication in relapse prevention in motivated opioid abusers (if users are not motivated, they will discontinue use). In the presence of naltrexone, opioids are ineffective (except with very high doses). While the use of naltrexone for opioid addiction is predictable, entirely unexpected was the finding that naltrexone was also effective in reducing alcohol consumption (Volpicelli, Alterman, Hayashida, & O'Brien, 1992). Such a finding indicates a clear link between alcohol use and endogenous opioid activity—and perhaps a common addiction pathway for alcohol and opioids, at a minimum.

NICOTINE

Just as methadone is used to treat opioid addiction, nicotine replacement therapy (gum, lozenge, nasal spray, patch) is used to facilitate smoking cessation. Although nicotine is the reinforcing chemical that drives smoking behavior, it is not the basis of the health problems related to cigarette use. The delivery vehicle for getting nicotine into the brain via the bloodstream—the cigarette—is loaded with plant chemicals that, when reduced to ashes, produce carcinogenic chemicals and raise circulating carbon monoxide levels. The consequence of this substance use disorder is that it dramatically increases the user's risk for developing lung damage (emphysema, cancer) and heart disease. The cost to both the user and society is high and smoking is becoming increasingly unacceptable to society (remember, abuse is a sociological not a pharmacological issue).

Nicotine replacement therapy, first of all, removes the carcinogens and the other harmful chemicals from the picture and allows the health care provider to focus exclusively on the behavior associated with this powerful reinforcer. Again, the goal is to extinguish—in this case, quite literally—the behavior. Nicotine replacement in the absence of behavioral therapy, therefore, will not work.

Bupropion is used clinically as an antidepressant (Wellbutrin) and for smoking cessation (Zyban). Bupropion blocks both dopamine and norepinephrine reuptake from neurons (see Chapter 2) and it is a nicotinic receptor antagonist. Although bupropion's action in smoking cessation can be entirely explained by its action on nicotine receptors, its action on DA reuptake may play a role as well since nicotine has been shown to increase extracellular DA in the nucleus accumbens. Bupropion reduces the severity of nicotine cravings and withdrawal symptoms. The efficacy of bupropion is similar to that of nicotine replacement therapy. Bupropion approximately doubles the chance of quitting smoking successfully after three months of use.

Varenicline (Chantix) is a high-affinity, partial agonist at the nicotinic acetylcholine receptor in the brain (Jorenby et al., 2006). As with buprenorphine and the opioids, the underlying hypothesis is that a partial agonist will facilitate abstinence by minimizing withdrawal symptoms yet will not be as reinforcing as the full agonist—in this case, nicotine. As such, the behavior extinguishes. In a direct comparison, varenicline (Chantix) showed superior efficacy to bupropion (Zyban) after one year. For placebo, the rate of abstinence was 10%, for bupropion it was 15%, and for varenicline it reached 23% (Jorenby et al., 2006).

ALCOHOL

One of the first drugs approved by the FDA to treat alcoholism was disulfiram (Antabuse). Consuming alcohol while taking disulfiram can cause the person to become violently ill. As such, disulfiram is a form of aversion therapy used to prevent relapse (Sadock, Kaplan, & Sadock, 2008). Alcohol is metabolized in the body in a two-step process. Ethanol is first metabolized by alcohol dehydrogenase to form acetaldehyde, which is subsequently metabolized by aldehyde dehydrogenase to generate acetic acid and water. Disulfiram inhibits the second enzyme, causing acetaldehyde to accumulate. This results in elevated skin temperature, facial flushing, rapid respiration and heart rate, lowered blood pressure, narrowing of the airways, nausea, and headache.

Several studies have shown disulfiram to decrease cocaine cravings (Table 7-10), even in patients who did not consume alcohol (Kampman, 2008). It turns out that disulfiram not only blocks aldehyde dehydrogenase, it also inhibits dopamine beta-hydroxylase, blocking the metabolism of cocaine and dopamine. Although counterintuitive—it seems like it would cause greater pleasure and increased use—it is believed that the high levels lead to increased anxiety and paranoia rather than euphoria. A recent clinical case report supports this hypothesis (Mutschler, Diehl, & Kiefer, 2009).

Acamprosate (Campral) is structurally related to GABA, and for many years it was assumed that its effectiveness in reducing alcohol consumption was due to the drug acting at the $GABA_A$ receptor. However, later studies showed that acamprosate does not bind to $GABA_A$ receptors or enhance their function, although it may inhibit $GABA_B$ autoreceptors (Gass & Olive, 2008). Acamprosate is an antagonist at NMDA (and other) glutamatergic receptors (Anton & Swift, 2003; Qatari, Bouchenafa, & Littleton, 1998) or via a combination of GABA activation and GLU blockade to reestablish their balance, which is disturbed by chronic alcohol exposure (Gass & Olive, 2008).

STIMULANTS

To date, there are no FDA-approved drugs on the market to treat stimulant (amphetamine, methamphetamine, cocaine) addiction or abuse. Many, many drugs have been tried for this purpose, none with clear, unambiguous success. Of the drugs being tested for this purpose (Table 7-10), all seem to work via one of three neurotransmitters: DA (disulfiram, aripiprazole), GLU (modafinil, memantine, lamotrigine, topirimate), or GABA (gabapentin, tiagabine).

Aripiprazole (Abilify) was approved by the FDA in 2002 for the treatment of *schizophrenia*, and more recently for treatment of acute manic and mixed episodes associated with *bipolar disorder*, and as an adjunct in the treatment of major depressive disorder (see Chapters 2, 3, and 4). Aripiprazole is a partial agonist at both the D_2 and 5-HT$_1$ receptors as well as an antagonist at the 5-HT$_{2A}$ receptor. The rationale for using a partial dopamine receptor agonist to treat stimulant addiction is the same as that for using buprenorphine (Subutex, Suboxone) to treat opioid addiction and varenicline (Chantix) for nicotine addiction. That is, it stimulates the receptors sufficiently to facilitate withdrawal and reduce cravings but not enough to be toxic or to be a drug of abuse itself. Early clinical trials suggest that it is at least partially effective in reducing cravings for both cocaine and amphetamine (Lile et al., 2005; Preti, 2007) but further studies are needed.

Given the prime role that GLU plays in excitatory neurotransmission, and the interactivity between DA and GLU (Table 7-8), it is not surprising that a number of drugs that work via GLU would be investigated for stimulant abuse. The inhibitory neurotransmitter GABA also acts on the nucleus accumbens (Hyman & Malenka, 2001). This would explain the keen interest in evaluating drugs that alter GABA neurotransmission for their effect on DA release in this region as well.

At this point a wide variety of drugs are in various phases of clinical trials (Phase I through Phase IV) to treat stimulant addiction although none have been FDA approved for clinical use (Preti, 2007).

THE MEANING OF ADDICTION

Most patients use opioids to control physical pain, but others use them to tamp down emotional pain or for a euphoric effect. Most patients use benzodiazepines to reduce anxiety or to help with sleep, but other people use them for disinhibition euphoria. Most patients use psychostimulants to manage ADHD or narcolepsy, but other people use them to produce a sense of exhilaration, improve self esteem, expand mental and physical performance, increase activity, diminish hunger, or stay awake longer.

These drugs and others have multiple effects, some good (therapeutic) and some bad (adverse). Here the adverse effect is addiction. But what is addiction? This was the original question posed at the beginning of this chapter. According to the American Psychiatric Association (APA) as codified most recently in DSM-IV-TR (American Psychiatric Association, 2000), the word *addiction* is no longer part of the professional lexicon[7]. Why, then, are there thousands of articles, hundreds of books, and dozens of journals containing this word?

Addiction is word that defines a pattern of behaviors that often do not involve drugs. The object may be food, gambling, shoplifting, or sex. Certain behaviors are always involved in addiction. These involve compulsive and impulsive actions, and these behaviors are difficult for a person to control despite the consequences. Perhaps the best definition of addiction is one by Goodman (2008):

> . . . addiction is a condition in which a behavior that can function both to produce pleasure and to reduce painful affects is employed in a pattern that is characterized by two key features: (1) recurrent failure to control the behavior, and (2) continuation of the behavior despite significant harmful consequences.

Perhaps the authors now in the late stage of planning of DSM-V will consider bringing back the word addiction. In the meantime, clinical and basic researchers throughout the world will continue their search for the magic bullet or bullets to defeat addiction.

---

[7]O'Brien (O'Brien, Volkow, & Li, 2006) notes that the decision to replace the word *addiction* with *dependence* passed by just one vote in the committee that developed the guidelines and that it was done because the word dependence was more neutral than addiction, which carried stigma.

REVIEW QUESTIONS

1. Is the following statement true or false? A synonym for an abused substance is a psychoactive drug.
   a. True
   b. False

2. Is the following statement true or false? Cocaine is a narcotic.
   a. True
   b. False
   c. Depends on your profession

3. Which of the following drugs was legally available in the United States at one time without a prescription?
   a. Heroin
   b. Amphetamine
   c. Cocaine
   d. All of the above

4. Which psychologist proposed that "a behavior followed by a reinforcing stimulus results in an increased probability of that behavior occurring in the future."
   a. Thomas Sydenham
   b. Wilhelm Sertürner
   c. Charles Bradley
   d. B. F. Skinner

5. Which of the following is a receptor for endogenous (e.g., endorphins) or exogenous (morphine) opioids?
   a. MOP (Mu, μ)
   b. D_2
   c. GABA$_A$
   d. NMDA

6. Which of the following drugs is most likely to be abused to attain "disinhibition euphoria"?
   a. Morphine
   b. Diazepam (Valium)
   c. Methylphenidate (Ritalin)
   d. Amphetamine(s) (Adderall)

7. What percent of children (6 to 17 years of age) and adults are estimated to have ADHD (or ADD)?
   a. 50% children; 50% adults
   b. 1% children; 10% adults
   c. 8% children; 4% adults
   d. 20% children; 0% adults

8. Which two neurotransmitters have been proposed as common links in addiction, regardless of the substance to which the person is addicted?
   a. Acetylcholine and GABA
   b. Endorphins and epinephrine
   c. Serotonin and histamine
   d. Dopamine and glutamate

9. Which of the following drugs used to facilitate discontinuation of usage and/or prevention of relapse is correctly paired with the drug of abuse for which the FDA has approved it?
   a. Buprenorphine (Suboxone) and cocaine
   b. Naltrexone (ReVia) and ethanol
   c. Varenicline (Chantix) and heroin
   d. Disulfiram (Antabuse) and nicotine

10. A(n) _____ is a drug used for the treatment of psychological, emotional, or behavior disorders.
    a. analgesic
    b. psychotherapeutic
    c. psychosomatic
    d. antiarrhythmic

REFERENCES

American Psychiatric Association. (2000). *Diagnostic and statistical manual of mental disorders: DSM-IV-TR.* (4th ed.). Washington, DC: American Psychiatric Association.

Anton, R. F., & Swift, R. M. (2003). Current pharmacotherapies of alcoholism: A U.S. perspective. *American Journal on Addictions, 12*(Suppl 1), S53–S68.

Barnard, E. A., Skolnick, P., Olsen, R. W., Mohler, H., Sieghart, W., Biggio, G., et al. (1998). International Union of Pharmacology. XV. Subtypes of gamma-aminobutyric acidA receptors: Classification on the basis of subunit structure and receptor function. *Pharmacological Reviews, 50*(2), 291–313.

Bodkin, J. A., Zornberg, G. L., Lukas, S. E., & Cole, J. O. (1995). Buprenorphine treatment of refractory depression. *Journal of Clinical Psychopharmacology, 15*(1), 49–57.

Bradley, C. B. (1937). The behavior of children receiving benzedrine. *American Journal of Psychiatry, 94*(3), 577–585.

Cerda, M., Sagdeo, A., & Galea, S. (2008). Comorbid forms of psychopathology: Key patterns and future research directions. *Epidemiologic Reviews, 30*, 155–177.

Corbett, A. D., Henderson, G., McKnight, A. T., & Paterson, S. J. (2006). 75 years of opioid research: The exciting but vain quest for the holy grail. *British Journal of Pharmacology, 147 Suppl 1*, S153–62.

Di Chiara, G. (1999). Drug addiction as dopamine-dependent associative learning disorder. *European Journal of Pharmacology, 375*(1–3), 13–30.

Esch, T., & Stefano, G. B. (2004). The neurobiology of pleasure, reward processes, addiction and their health implications. *Neuroendocrinology Letters, 25*(4), 235–251.

Fainsinger, R. L., Thai, V., Frank, G., & Fergusson, J. (2006). What's in a word? Addiction versus dependence in DSM-V. *American Journal of Psychiatry, 163*(11), 2014.

Findling, R. L. (2008). Evolution of the treatment of attention-deficit/hyperactivity disorder in children: A review. *Clinical Therapeutics, 30*(5), 942–957.

Gass, J. T., & Olive, M. F. (2008). Glutamatergic substrates of drug addiction and alcoholism. *Biochemical Pharmacology, 75*(1), 218–265.

Goodman, A. (2008). Neurobiology of addiction. An integrative review. *Biochemical Pharmacology, 75*(1), 266–322.

Hyman, S. E., & Malenka, R. C. (2001). Addiction and the brain: The neurobiology of compulsion and its persistence. *Nature Reviews Neuroscience, 2*(10), 695–703.

Jorenby, D. E., Hays, J. T., Rigotti, N. A., Azoulay, S., Watsky, E. J., Williams, K. E., et al. (2006). Efficacy of varenicline, an alpha4beta2 nicotinic acetylcholine receptor partial agonist, vs placebo or sustained-release bupropion for smoking cessation: A randomized controlled trial. *JAMA: The Journal of the American Medical Association, 296*(1), 56–63.

Kampman, K. M. (2008). The search for medications to treat stimulant dependence. *Addiction Science & Clinical Practice, 4*(2), 28–35.

Krambeer, L. L., von McKnelly, W., Jr., Gabrielli, W. F., Jr., & Penick, E. C. (2001). Methadone therapy for opioid dependence. *American Family Physician, 63*(12), 2404–2410.

Kessler, R. C., Adler, L., Barkley, R., Biederman, J., Conners, C. K., Demler, O., et al. (2006). The prevalence and correlates of adult ADHD in the United States: Results from the National Comorbidity Survey replication. *American Journal of Psychiatry, 163*(4), 716–723.

Lile, J. A., Stoops, W. W., Vansickel, A. R., Glaser, P. E., Hays, L. R., & Rush, C. R. (2005). Aripiprazole attenuates the discriminative-stimulus and subject-rated effects of D-amphetamine in humans. *Neuropsychopharmacology, 30*(11), 2103–2114.

Lydiard, R. B. (2003). The role of GABA in anxiety disorders. *Journal of Clinical Psychiatry, 64*(Suppl 3), 21–27.

Markowitz, J. S., & Patrick, K. S. (2008). Differential pharmacokinetics and pharmacodynamics of methylphenidate enantiomers: Does chirality matter? *Journal of Clinical Psychopharmacology, 28*(3 Suppl 2), S54–S61.

McCann, D. J. (2008). Potential of buprenorphine/naltrexone in treating polydrug addiction and co-occurring psychiatric disorders. *Clinical Pharmacology & Therapeutics, 83*(4), 627–630.

McGough, J. J., Pataki, C. S., & Suddath, R. (2005). Dexmethylphenidate extended-release capsules for attention deficit hyperactivity disorder. *Expert Review of Neurotherapeutics, 5*(4), 437–441.

Mollereau, C., & Mouledous, L. (2000). Tissue distribution of the opioid receptor-like (ORL1) receptor. *Peptides, 21*(7), 907–917.

Mutschler, J., Diehl, A., & Kiefer, F. (2009). Pronounced paranoia as a result of cocaine-disulfiram interaction: Case report and mode of action. *Journal of Clinical Psychopharmacology, 29*(1), 99–101.

National Institute on Drug Abuse. (2009). *NIDA drugs of abuse and related topics - media guide.* Retrieved 5/31/2009, 2009, from http://www.drugabuse.gov/mediaguide/scienceof.html

National Institutes of Health. *A double-blind study of buprenorphine treatment of acute suicidality—ClinicalTrials.gov.* Retrieved 6/4/2009, 2009, from http://clinicaltrials.gov/ct2/show/NCT00863291

National Institutes of Health. (2009). *Principles of drug addiction treatment: A research based guide.* National Institutes of Health.

O'Brien, C. P., Volkow, N., & Li, T. K. (2006). What's in a word? addiction versus dependence in DSM-V. *American Journal of Psychiatry, 163*(5), 764–765.

Olsen, R. W., & Sieghart, W. (2008). International union of pharmacology. LXX. Subtypes of gamma-aminobutyric acid(A) receptors: Classification on the basis of subunit composition, pharmacology, and function. Update. *Pharmacological Reviews, 60*(3), 243–260.

Pastor, P. N. (2008). *Diagnosed attention deficit hyperactivity disorder and learning disability, United States, 2004–2006: Data from the National Health Interview Survey (DHHS Publication).* Centers for Disease Control and Prevention. http://www.cdc.gov/nchs/data/series/sr_10/sr10_237.pdf

Patrick, K. S., Williard, R. L., VanWert, A. L., Dowd, J. J., Oatis, J. E., Jr., & Middaugh, L. D. (2005). Synthesis and pharmacology of ethylphenidate enantiomers: The human transesterification metabolite of methylphenidate and ethanol. *Journal of Medicinal Chemistry, 48*(8), 2876–2881.

Pert, C. B., & Snyder, S. H. (1973). Opiate receptor: Demonstration in nervous tissue. *Science, 179*(77), 1011–1014.

Preti, A. (2007). New developments in the pharmacotherapy of cocaine abuse. *Addiction Biology, 12*(2), 133–151.

Qatari, M., Bouchenafa, O., & Littleton, J. (1998). Mechanism of action of acamprosate. Part II. Ethanol dependence modifies effects of acamprosate on NMDA receptor binding in membranes from rat cerebral cortex. *Alcoholism Clinical and Experimental Research, 22*(4), 810.

Quello, S. B., Brady, K. T., & Sonne, S. C. (2005). Mood disorders and substance use disorder: A complex comorbidity. *Science & Practice Perspectives : A Publication of the National Institute on Drug Abuse, National Institutes of Health, 3*(1), 13–21.

Robinson, T. E., & Berridge, K. C. (1993). The neural basis of drug craving: An incentive-sensitization theory of addiction. *Brain Research—Brain Research Reviews, 18*(3), 247–291.

Robinson, T. E., & Kolb, B. (2004). Structural plasticity associated with exposure to drugs of abuse. *Neuropharmacology, 47*(Suppl 1), 33–46.

Sadock, B. J., Kaplan, H. I., & Sadock, V. A. (2008). Biological therapies. *Kaplan & Sadock's concise textbook of clinical psychiatry.* Philadelphia: Wolters Kluwer/Lippincott Williams & Wilkins.

SAMHSA, Office of Applied Studies. (2009). *Results from the 2008 National Survey on Drug Use and Health: National findings, SAMHSA, OAS.* Retrieved 1/31/2010, from http://oas.samhsa.gov/nsduh/2k8nsduh/2k8Results.pdf

Skinner, B. F. (1938). *The behavior of organisms: An experimental analysis.* Englewood Cliffs, NJ: Prentice-Hall.

Srivastava, A., & Kahan, M. (2006). Buprenorphine: A potential new treatment option for opioid dependence. *CMAJ: Canadian Medical Association Journal—Journal De l'Association Medicale Canadienne, 174*(13), 1835.

Szumlinski, K. K., Ary, A. W., & Lominac, K. D. (2008). Homers regulate drug-induced neuroplasticity: Implications for addiction. *Biochemical Pharmacology, 75*(1), 112–133.

Szumlinski, K. K., Kalivas, P. W., & Worley, P. F. (2006). Homer proteins: Implications for neuropsychiatric disorders. *Current Opinion in Neurobiology, 16*(3), 251–257.

Quinton, The Rt. Hon. Lord., The Oxford Companion to Philosophy. (2005). *"Philosopher's Stone" Oxford Reference Online.* Retrieved 6/2/2009, 2009, from http://www.oxfordreference.com/views/ENTRY.html?subview=Main&entry=t116.e1905

U.S. Department of Justice, Drug Enforcement Administration. *Section 802: Title 21 United States Code (USC) Controlled Substances Act.* Retrieved 5/31/2009, 2009, from http://www.deadiversion.usdoj.gov/21cfr/21usc/802.htm

Uys, J. D., & LaLumiere, R. T. (2008). Glutamate: The new frontier in pharmacotherapy for cocaine addiction. *CNS & Neurological Disorders Drug Targets, 7*(5), 482–491.

Volpicelli, J. R., Alterman, A. I., Hayashida, M., & O'Brien, C. P. (1992). Naltrexone in the treatment of alcohol dependence. *Archives of General Psychiatry, 49*(11), 876–880.

ANSWER KEY

CHAPTER 1

1. d. Physiology is the science of the normal functions and phenomena of living organisms. Neurophysiology is the study of the nervous system.

2. d. The lowest level of the brain is the brainstem, above which is the cerebellum, topped by the forebrain.

3. d. The cortex has already processed sensory information the hippocampus receives. Extended (about a year), but not permanent, memory of facts and events is regulated by the hippocampus and damage to it can affect memory storage.

4. a. The neurological disorder Parkinson's disease is due to a degeneration of dopamine-producing cell bodies in the substantia nigra with fibers that terminate in the basal nuclei. Damage to this pathway interferes with fine-tuned motor function needed for most common motor functions.

5. b. The raphe nuclei are located at the junction of the pons and the medulla. Many neurons here secrete 5-HT and send fibers to innervate the diencephalon and cerebral cortex. Other fibers descend to the spinal cord and may be involved in pain pathways.

6. c. The hypothalamus is a unique junction in the brain. The hypothalamus receives and transmits information via both neurons and hormones. Neuronal information from higher areas of the brain triggers the hypothalamus to release several hormones.

7. b. The advantage of all the folding in the brain is that it allows a larger surface area to exist in a tightly contained solid chamber (the skull). The cerebral cortex contains about 50 to 60 billion neurons and makes about 240 trillion synapses.

8. c. All of the statements are correct except c. Acetylcholine is an excitatory transmitter. The most abundant excitatory transmitter in the nervous system is glutamate (GLU).

9. d. Both the mesolimbic and the mesocortical dopamine pathways play critical roles in the brain's reward and pleasure centers. Drugs that elevate dopamine levels in these areas of the brain (cocaine, amphetamines) have a high potential for abuse.

10. a. THC appears to exert its effects by acting on receptors for endocannabinoids. The pathway regulates such diverse physiological processes as learning, memory, appetite control, and reward, as well as certain pathological processes such as pain, anxiety, and mood disorders.

CHAPTER 2

1. c. The goal of treatment with an antidepressant is full recovery, in which the patient is symptom free for at least one year. Until then, if patients have no symptoms, they are said to be in remission. Relapse occurs if symptoms of depression recur before the "anniversary," and recurrence is when symptoms return after recovery has taken place (>1 year of remission).

2. c. The MAHOD was an early, overly simple explanation for how antidepressants and antimanic drugs would work. It was also incorrect. The biggest problem is timing. If a deficiency in some aspect of monoamine (NE, DA, or 5-HT) was responsible for depression, then raising their levels (which happens with TCAs, MAOIs, and SSRIs) should produce immediate (within a day) symptom relief. But they don't, nullifying this theory.

3. c. Often, after a drug is introduced, other uses may be discovered. To minimize confusion, drug companies may market the same generic drug with different trade names. Bupropion is an excellent example. It is sold as Wellbutrin when used for depression and as Zyban when sold for smoking cessation. Similarly, when used for hypertension, minoxidil is sold as Loniten, and as Rogaine when used for hair regrowth.

4. a. The most challenging clinical problem today for pharmaceutical companies and researchers is to find an antidepressant that is safe and rapid acting. While today antidepressants are far safer that the TCAs and MAOIs, they do not work any faster, a minimum of 10 to 14 days is needed before clinical improvement is seen. Small clinical trials with ketamine promise a potential new treatment direction in which antidepressants might have a more immediate onset.

5. b. Neurotrophic factors, in general, are chemical substances in the brain that guide nervous system development. Recent studies indicate that neurotrophic factors such as BDNF play a critical role in the adult brain, as well. In theory a lack of brain BDNF would allow certain vulnerable neurons in the hippocampus to atrophy and die, engendering the signs and symptoms of depression.

6.

Frontal cortex (d)	a. orgasm and ejaculation
Basal nuclei (c)	b. appetite and eating behavior
Hypothalamus (b)	c. movement
Spinal cord (a)	d. mood

Axons originating in neurons from the raphe nucleus project to several areas of the brain and regulate physiological functions and behaviors. Axons from the raphe nucleus project to the frontal cortex, which regulates mood; the basal nuclei, which helps control movements as well as obsessions and compulsions; the limbic system, which appears to be involved in anxiety and panic; the hypothalamus, which regulates (among many other functions) appetite and eating behavior; the brainstem, which regulates sleep; and the spinal cord, which controls several reflexes involved in normal sexual response (orgasm and ejaculation).

7. b. In areas of the brain, such as the hippocampus, BDNF is needed to maintain normal function. BDNF levels are diminished in depression, an effect that can be reversed by all clinically effective antidepressants. In the absence of BDNF, brain cells die (apoptosis), neuroplasticity is diminished (cognitive dysfunction), and neurogenesis is diminished (no new brain cells replace the ones that die). In the presence of BDNF hippocampal cells sprout and recovery occurs.

8. c. The major clinical advantage of using SSRIs and newer antidepressants is the reduced incidence of life-threatening adverse effects associated with the older drugs, most of which were due to their actions on NE, 5-HT, ACh, and other receptors. These newer drugs are not only safer for the patient but also allow the family physician or NP to directly treat the patient rather than have a psychiatrist manage the patient.

9. b. It appears that elevating both NE and 5-HT levels, through the use of two drugs or a single drug that acts by both mechanisms, such as venlafaxine, may be beneficial when a single drug alone is not effective.

10. d. Clinical studies with ketamine suggest that a rapid onset antidepressant may be available in the near future. Ketamine may not be the right drug because it can produce severe nightmares and hallucinations, but it suggests a new direction of research for antidepressant drug development, by blocking the NMDA subtype of the glutamate receptor in brain.

CHAPTER 3

1. c. At one time bipolar patients were treated with lithium during acute manic episodes and prophylactically during euthymic periods. When depressed, these patients were treated with traditional antidepressants, such as MAOIs, TCAs, and, later, SSRIs. Often, these patients would rapidly switch moods and became acutely manic. Today, to prevent this from happening, it is common for bipolar patients to be kept on a mood stabilizer at all times, even when taking an antidepressant concurrently.

2. a. Three classes of drugs are commonly used as mood stabilizers in bipolar patients. Lithium, for many years, was the only such drug available. Today, in addition to lithium, a subset of anticonvulsants are effective as mood stabilizers. These include valproic acid, carbamazepine, and lamotrigine. Others are not effective, and newer drugs have not been adequately tested. Antipsychotics, particularly the newer atypical or second-generation drugs have been shown to be clinically effective as well.

3. b. A very specific single nucleotide polymorphism (SNP) occurs in the genetic formula for the BDNF precursor protein in certain individuals. Even though the portion of the precursor molecule where this occurs is snipped off before the final BDNF protein is synthesized, it, nonetheless, can affect BDNF release and can affect behavior. Several studies suggest that individuals with the Val66Val form may have a higher incidence of early-onset and rapid-cycling bipolar disorder. However, those with the Val66Met or Met66Met form may have issues related to learning and memory.

4. e. All of the above treatments, including lithium, SSRIs, TCAs, and electroconvulsive therapy can increase hippocampal BDNF levels.

5. d. The above symptoms describe cyclothymia, a milder form of bipolar, which may be difficult to diagnose. First-line treatment usually involves a mood stabilizer such as lithium, an anticonvulsant, or an atypical antipsychotic. Although an antidepressant may be used, as with other bipolar disorders, it should not be used alone, for fear of triggering a rapid mood reversal (severe manic episode).

6. b. Although several brain structures may be affected in mood disorders, two key structures are the hippocampus and the frontal cortex. The hippocampus is part of the limbic system. The frontal cortex is part of the cerebral hemisphere. Disturbances in these regions appear to account for most of the cognitive and behavioral symptoms of mood disorders.

7. d. In general, the less often patients need to take a drug, the better is their compliance. This is true for venlafaxine, a drug whose short plasma half-life is dealt with by packaging it in a slow or extended release formulation. In this manner, it can be taken once daily. Moreover, one of the most common adverse effects of venlafaxine, nausea, is greatly reduced in the extended (slow) release formulation as the blood level rises only gradually after each dose.

8. a. While the newer antidepressants have overcome one of the major stumbling blocks in treating depressed patients—the TCAs and MAOIs are very toxic, with low therapeutic indices—they still do not act rapidly. All clinically useful antidepressants take 10 to 60 days to achieve clinical effectiveness, if they work at all. While newer drugs are safer than the older antidepressants, none work any faster and some may actually be less efficacious.

9. b. Bipolar I and bipolar II differ in several respects including the severity of the two primary symptoms, depression and mania. For bipolar I patients, the intense manic episodes may require hospitalization to bring under control. For bipolar II patients, the depressive symptoms dominate and, when hospitalization is needed, it is usually for this reason (e.g., attempted suicide or suicidal thoughts). Since some patients may display characteristics of depression and mania simultaneously (i.e., mixed episode), the DSM category Bipolar-NOS (not otherwise specified) has been developed.

10. a. Cade first reported the clinical effectiveness of lithium, in 1949. He found it to be effective in all 10 manic patients he treated but ineffective in any of his patients with dementia praecox (schizophrenia). Later it was found to be effective not only in treating acute mania, but also prophylactically, in preventing mood swings in either direction. Because of its low therapeutic index, other drugs have been used when lithium cannot tolerated by a patient.

CHAPTER 4

1. a. Although FGAs revolutionized the treatment of psychotic patients, they were most effective against the positive symptoms of the disorder. In addition, because all FGAs blocked all D_2 receptors, even in areas of the brain in which function was presumed to be normal (e.g., the caudate nucleus in the striatum), they all caused motor problems (pseudoparkinsonism). SGAs have a much lower incidence of motor impairments and can help reduce the negative and cognitive symptoms of schizophrenia better that the FGAs.

2. d. The mesolimbic pathway runs from the tegmentum in the midbrain to nucleus accumbens in the limbic system. It is believed to mediate the positive symptoms of schizophrenia. This is where FGAs are believed to exert their therapeutic action. Blockade of the other three DA pathways in the brain may actually contribute toward the adverse effects of FGAs.

3. b. There is little doubt that clozapine would be the drug of first choice in treating schizophrenia if it did not produce the potentially lethal adverse effect, agranulocytosis.

4. d. Weight gain during treatment is a common problem with SGAs and is often the basis for poor compliance. The ADA recommends a change in drug if the patient gains more than 5% of baseline weight while taking the drugs. In addition, the incidence of new-onset type 2 diabetes may be as high as 52% with SGAs and blood lipid levels are significantly elevated as well. These changes may be associated with a higher incidence of myocarditis and cardiomyopathies.

5. b. Although Hofmann and other scientists of his time held out hope that LSD might be useful to help understand the underlying basis of schizophrenia and other psychiatric disorders, the drug never fulfilled this promise and became nothing more (and nothing less) than a recreational drug. Two key differences between the hallucinations caused by LSD and those experienced by schizophrenic patients are: (1) LSD hallucinations were visual whereas in schizophrenia they are primarily auditory in nature, and (2) LSD users are keenly aware that they are in an altered state, whereas schizophrenic patients think they are normal. Had Dr. Hofmann studied amphetamine or cocaine-induced psychosis, he might have been more successful in his endeavors to find a drug model for schizophrenia.

6. d. The four major dopamine (DA) pathways in the brain are believed to be responsible for the therapeutic and adverse effects of all first- and most second-generation antipsychotics. Other neurotransmitters, such as 5-HT, GLU, and GABA may also be involved in schizophrenia. The four DA pathways are the mesolimbic, mesocortical, nigrostriatal, and tuberoinfundibular (from the hypothalamus to the anterior pituitary) pathways.

7. c. Although clozapine may be the single most effective antipsychotic, because of the relatively high incidence of the potentially fatal adverse effect, agranulocytosis, it is not the drug of first choice for most schizophrenic patients.

8. d. The second-generation antipsychotic medications are the treatments of choice for schizophrenia

in older patients, due to a lower risk of both extrapyramidal side effects and tardive dyskinesia.

9. c. SGAs are, more often than not, the drugs of first choice in treating schizophrenia. These drugs are less likely than the FGAs to produce EPS or pseudoparkinsonism symptoms. Whereas all FGAs act by blocking DA receptors, SGAs also block 5-HT receptors.

10. d. DA, released by the tuberoinfundibular pathway, which is from the hypothalamus to the pituitary gland, inhibits prolactin release. Blockade of this pathway by FGAs can lead to prolactinemia and the symptoms above.

CHAPTER 5

1. a. While ADHD was once thought to occur in childhood only, it is now known that it continues into adolescence in about 60% to 80% of patients and remains a problem in adulthood in as many as 30% to 40% of patients.

2. a. Three of the four brain pathways believed to be involved in the mechanism of action of drugs used to treat ADHD have DA as their neurotransmitter (mesocortical, nigrostriatal, and mesolimbic). Only one pathway (prefrontal) utilizes NE. This pathway affects areas of the brain involved in sustaining and focusing attention, maintaining motivation, and in working memory.

3. d. All traditional drugs used to treat ADHD (i.e., amphetamines and methylphenidate) have abuse potential and are DEA Schedule II controlled substances. Atomoxetine is a selective NE reuptake inhibitor with no abuse potential.

4. a. Memory problems in AD patients coincide with neuronal loss in the NBM. Within approximately three years, as cell damage and loss spreads to areas of the brain receiving cholinergic innervation from the NBM (e.g., hippocampus and amygdala, cerebral cortex), the patient loses functional independence and an early diagnosis of AD can be made. Three to six years later, the neocortex is heavily involved in the disease process and the patient generally needs to be placed into a nursing home to assure proper care. With few exceptions these patients die over the ensuing three years.

5. c. Because the drugs currently used to treat AD all increase acetylcholine levels throughout the brain and body (by blocking its metabolism), these drugs have many adverse effects (e.g., nausea, anorexia, vomiting, and diarrhea) that limit the maximal dose that can be used to treat AD patients.

6. d. The mesolimbic pathway, from the ventral tegmentum to the nucleus accumbens is involved the pleasurable effects (i.e., euphoria) produced by the psychostimulant drugs and is the basis of their abuse liability.

7. d. The major advantage of these preparations is that they can be given only once per day and do not have to be administered during school hours. Even though these drugs have durations of action of 12 hours or less, they are not given a second (or third time) per day. Use later in the day would interfere with sleep.

8. a. Atomoxetine (Strattera), a highly selective NE reuptake inhibitor, is the only first-line ADHD medication that has no abuse potential and is not a DEA Schedule II controlled substance. It does not directly affect DA levels in the nucleus accumbens, the area of the brain that mediates the euphoric properties (i.e., abuse liability) of the psychostimulants. It is the only drug approved by the FDA to treat adult ADHD.

9. a. In AD patients, cholinergic neurons innervating the cerebral cortex develop neurofibrillary tangles, small twisted neurofilaments, and accumulate around the neuron's microtubules. In addition, on the exterior of NBM neurons, beta-amyloid polypeptides are overproduced and accumulate in the synapse.

10. a. All drugs used to treat the cognitive and memory problems of mild to moderate AD elevate acetylcholine (ACh) levels by inhibiting its degradative enzyme, acetylcholinesterase (AChE). As a class, they are referred to as cholinesterase inhibitors. All of the drugs, other than venlafaxine, are cholinesterase inhibitors. Although venlafaxine may be used to treat depression in AD patients, it is not used to help memory or cognitive dysfunction.

CHAPTER 6

CORRECT ANSWERS:

1.	Buspirone (BuSpar)	a.	5-HT
2.	Diazepam (Valium)	d.	GABA
3.	Propranolol (Inderal)	c.	Norepinephrine
4.	Ramelteon (Rozerem)	b.	Melatonin

Anxiety and insomnia may be treated with a number of different drugs acting through a variety of neurotransmitters. For some types of anxiety, drugs whose mechanism of action involves serotonin (buspirone) work best. With other types of anxiety, a norepinephrine-based mechanism (propranolol) is preferable and with others, drugs acting via GABA (diazepam) are ideal. Ramelteon (Rozerem) is an agonist at melatonin receptors in the suprachiasmatic nucleus (SCN) and is approved for long-term use in adults for sleep problems.

5. d. Many clinically useful drugs are agonists or antagonists at receptor binding sites for a particular neurotransmitter. The benzodiazepines, non-benzodiazepine benzodiazepine agonists (NBBAs), and the barbiturates bind to secondary binding sites on the $GABA_A$ receptor complex to produce their effects in the brain. In their presence, when GABA binds to its receptor, it is far more effective at opening chloride channels than in their absence.

6. b. Zaleplon is a NBBA that binds to the omega-1 subtype of the BZ receptor. This receptor subtype specificity allows zaleplon (and other NBBAs) to be used exclusively for insomnia. Unlike the BZs, these drugs are not anxiolytic and they cannot be used to prevent or relieve seizures.

7. c. Several dietary supplements and herbs are marketed to improve sleep health (not to treat insomnia). These include melatonin, valerian root, hops, kava, chamomile, and lemon balm.

8. d. Although, barbiturates developed in the early twentieth century, were safer than older drugs, they presented a host of problems that led to their replacement in the treatment of insomnia by benzodiazepines in the 1960s. Barbiturates are inducers of drug metabolism, which may lead to many drug interactions. Unlike the BZs, high doses of barbiturates depress all electrically excitable tissue including respiratory and cardiovascular systems. Moreover, low doses of barbiturates cannot be used to treat anxiety. The anxiolytic dose of barbiturates is always sedating, precluding the use of these drugs for that purpose. Today, the primary use of barbiturates is for the treatment of epilepsy (phenobarbital) and induction of anesthesia (thiopental).

9. d. Propranolol is particularly effective at blocking the noradrenergic signs of anxiety including tachycardia, dilated pupils, sweating, and tremor, which are mediated by the beta subtype of the receptor. The NE anxiolytics may be the drugs of choice for social phobias.

10. a. Almost all OTC sleep aids contain an antihistamine, most often diphenhydramine, which is the active ingredient in the allergy medication Benadryl.

CHAPTER 7

1. b. Although all drugs of abuse are psychoactive (i.e., they affect behavior), not all psychoactive drugs are abused. These are not synonymous terms. Certain drugs are abused because they produce a reinforcing stimulus (i.e., pleasure). When this occurs the behavior is more likely to be repeated. Thus, amphetamine is abused and venlafaxine (Effexor) is not.

2. c. Although no health care provider would ever refer to cocaine as a narcotic (it is a stimulant), under federal legal statutes (Section 802 of the United States Controlled Substances Act), cocaine is classified as a narcotic.

3. d. Before the high-abuse potentials of drugs were known or before society decided to restrict their use, many substances, currently regulated by the DEA, were available in the United States without a prescription. These include heroin (for coughs), cocaine for toothaches, and amphetamine for nasal congestion.

4. d. B. F. Skinner developed the idea that the probability of a behavior occurring again is determined by its consequences.

5. a. The four primary receptors for opioids are the MOP (Mu, μ), KOP (kappa, k), DOP (delta, d), and the NOP (nociceptin) subtypes. The D_2 receptors are for dopamine, $GABA_A$ is for gamma-amino butyric acid, and NMDA is a glutamate receptor subtype.

6. b. While each of these drugs may be abused, the benzodiazepines (and alcohol) are used to produce disinhibition euphoria, a pleasurable (and, therefore, able to be reinforced) sensation caused by the loss of inhibitions.

7. c. In the United States, ADHD is diagnosed in an approximately 8% of school-age children. ADHD is not just a childhood illness. The prevalence of ADHD in adults is about 4.4% and is directly proportional to the severity of ADHD in childhood.

8. d. While no single neurochemical has been shown to be the substrate of addiction, the two that have been most investigated and which have substantial clinical evidence in their favor are dopamine and glutamate.

9. b. Naltrexone (ReVia) has been FDA approved for use in the treatment of both opioid and alcohol addiction. Varenicline (Chantix) is approved to treat smoking cessation, disulfiram (Antabuse) for alcohol abuse, and buprenorphine (Suboxone) to reduce opioid cravings.

10. b. Psychotherapeutic or psychoactive drugs are used for the treatment of psychological, emotional, or behavior disorders.

ABBREVIATION LIST

α_1	Alpha-1 adrenergic		LTP	Long-term potentiation
5-HT	Serotonin (5-hydroxy tryptamine)		M	Muscarinic-cholinergic
A	Adenine		MAD	Mixed anxiety depression
ACh	Acetylcholine		MAHOD	Monoamine hypothesis of depression
AChE	Acetylcholinesterase		MAO	Monoamine oxidase
AD	Alzheimer's disease		MAOI	Monoamine oxidase inhibitors
ADHD	Attention deficit hyperactivity disorder		MC	Mesocortical DA pathway
AIMS	Abnormal involuntary movement scale		MDD	Major depressive disorder
AP	Action potential		ML	Mesolimbic DA pathway
ApoE	Apolipoprotein E		MPH	d,l-threo-methylphenidate
BDNF	Brain-derived neurotrophic factor		MRI	Magnetic resonance imaging
BuChE	Butyrylcholinesterase		NBBA	Non-BZ BZ-receptor agonist
BZ	Benzodiazepine		NBM	Nucleus basalis of Meynert
CB	Cannabinoid receptors		NE	Norepinephrine
ChAT	Choline acetyltransferase		NT	Neurotransmitter
CNS	Central nervous system		NS	Nigrostriatal DA pathway
CYP	Cytochrome P450		NO	Nitric oxide
D_2	D_2 subtype of dopamine receptor		NSAIDs	Non-steroidal anti-inflammatory drugs
DA	Dopamine		PNS	Peripheral nervous system
DSM-IV-TR	Diagnostic and Statistical Manual, 4th ed, Text Revision		ProBDNF	Protein for BDNF
ECT	Electroconvulsive therapy		RAS	Reticular activating system
EPS	Extrapyramidal symptoms		SCN	Suprachiasmatic nucleus
FGA	First generation antipsychotics		SGA	Second generation antipsychotics (atypical)
fMRI	Functional magnetic resonance imaging		SNP	Single nucleotide polymorphisms
G	Guanine		SNRI	Selective serotonin and norepinephrine reuptake inhibitors
GABA	Gamma-aminobutyric acid			
GAD	Generalized anxiety disorder		SSRI	Selective serotonin reuptake inhibitors
GLU	Glutamate		TCA	Tricyclic antidepressants
H_1	Histaminergic		TD	Tardivedyskinesia
LC	Locus ceruleus		TI	Tuberoinfundibular DA pathway
LDL	Low-density lipoproteins		VLDL	Very low-density lipoproteins
LSD	Lysergic acid diethylamide		VTA	Ventral tegmental area

INDEX

Note: Page numbers followed by f or t refer to Figures or Tables.